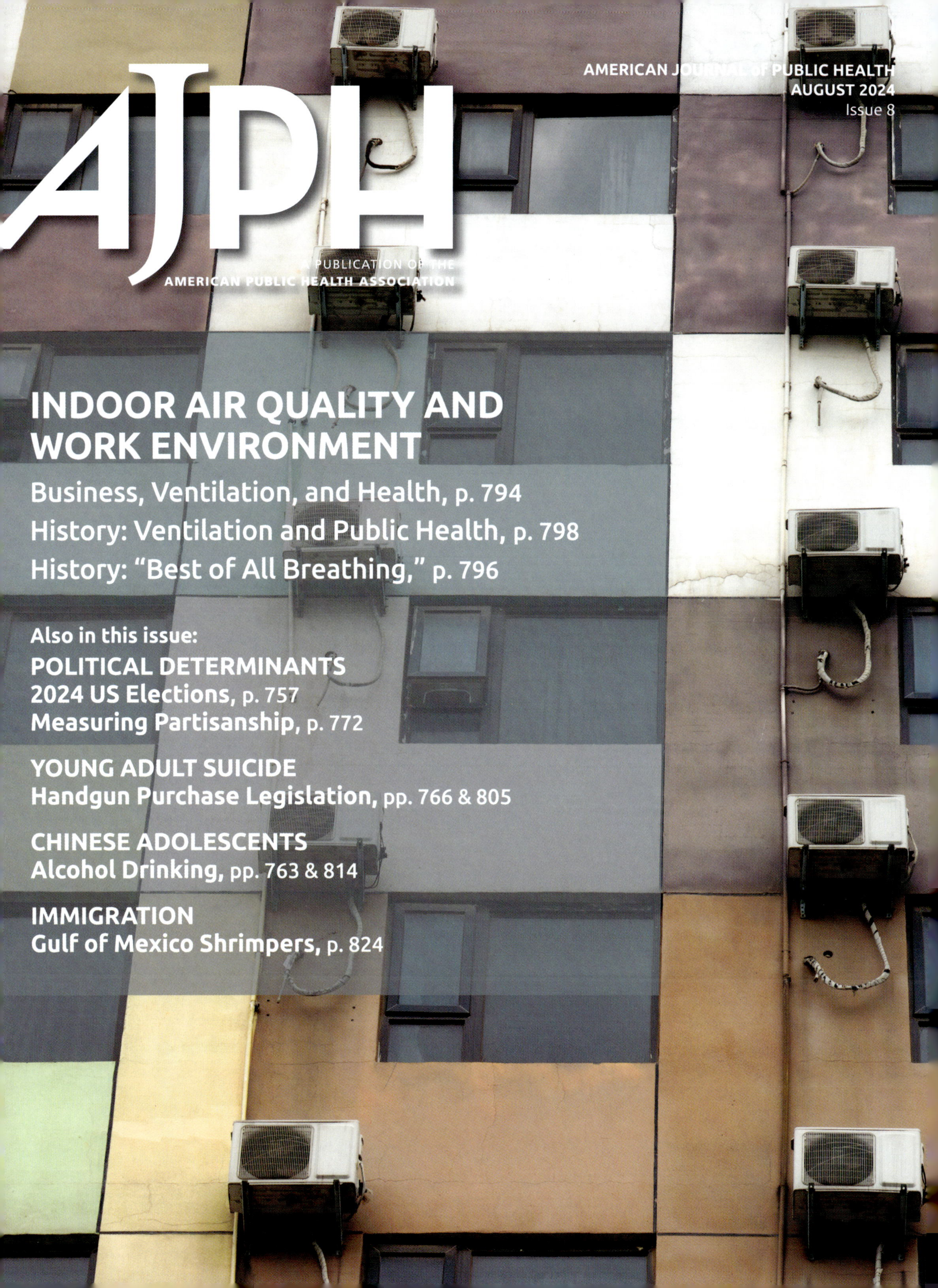

AJPH

A PUBLICATION OF THE
AMERICAN PUBLIC HEALTH ASSOCIATION

AMERICAN JOURNAL of PUBLIC HEALTH
AUGUST 2024
Issue 8

INDOOR AIR QUALITY AND WORK ENVIRONMENT

Business, Ventilation, and Health, p. 794

History: Ventilation and Public Health, p. 798

History: "Best of All Breathing," p. 796

Also in this issue:

POLITICAL DETERMINANTS
2024 US Elections, p. 757
Measuring Partisanship, p. 772

YOUNG ADULT SUICIDE
Handgun Purchase Legislation, pp. 766 & 805

CHINESE ADOLESCENTS
Alcohol Drinking, pp. 763 & 814

IMMIGRATION
Gulf of Mexico Shrimpers, p. 824

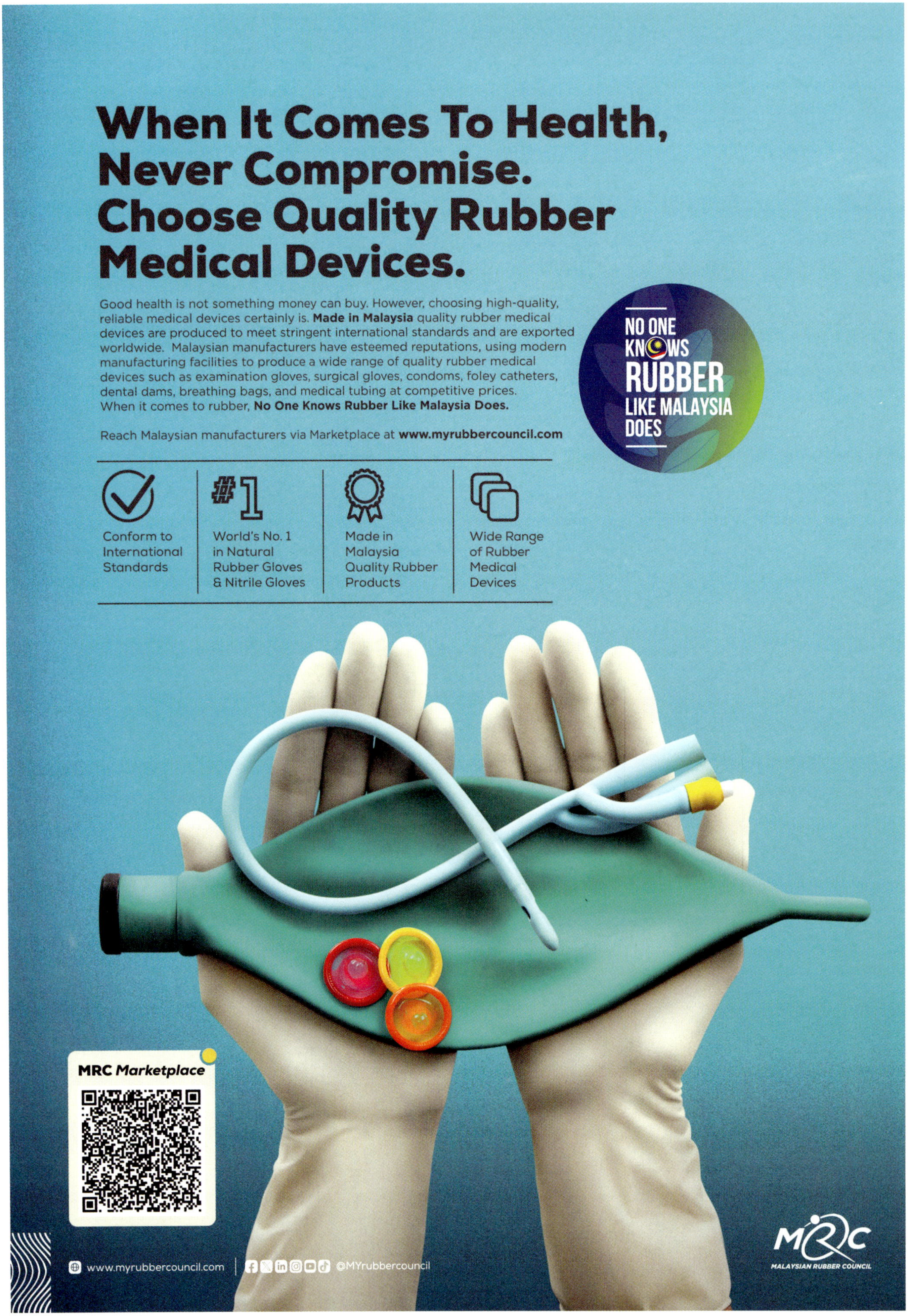
When It Comes To Health, Never Compromise. Choose Quality Rubber Medical Devices.
Good health is not something money can buy. However, choosing high-quality, reliable medical devices certainly is. Made in Malaysia quality rubber medical devices are produced to meet stringent international standards and are exported worldwide. Malaysian manufacturers have esteemed reputations, using modern manufacturing facilities to produce a wide range of quality rubber medical devices such as examination gloves, surgical gloves, condoms, foley catheters, dental dams, breathing bags, and medical tubing at competitive prices. When it comes to rubber, No One Knows Rubber Like Malaysia Does.
Reach Malaysian manufacturers via Marketplace at www.myrubbercouncil.com
NO ONE KNOWS RUBBER LIKE MALAYSIA DOES
Conform to International Standards
#1
World's No. 1 in Natural Rubber Gloves & Nitrile Gloves
Made in Malaysia Quality Rubber Products
Wide Range of Rubber Medical Devices
MRC Marketplace
www.myrubbercouncil.com
@MYrubbercouncil
MRC
MALAYSIAN RUBBER COUNCIL

APHA
AMERICAN PUBLIC HEALTH ASSOCIATION
For science. For action. For health.

AJPH®, published monthly, is the official Journal of the American Public Health Association®, 800 I St NW, Washington, DC 20001-3710; (202) 777- APHA; TDD (202) 777-2500. APHA is a nongovernmental professional society founded in 1872, representing all disciplines and specialties in public health.

The *American Journal of Public Health*® (*AJPH*) (print ISSN: 0090-0036; electronic ISSN: 1541- 0048), first published in 1911, is the official journal of the American Public Health Association® (APHA). The oldest and largest organization of public health professionals in the world, APHA represents approximately 30 000 members from more than 50 occupations of public health.

Submissions: Visit www.editorialmanager.com/ajph or ajph.edmgr.com for online manuscript preparation and submission guidelines. Contributions of original unpublished research, social science analyses, scholarly essays, critical commentaries, departments, and letters to the editor are welcome. Questions? Write ajph.submissions@apha.org or call APHA at (202) 777-2469.

Print plus online subscriptions: Institutional price (print copy with online access for a single institution and all authorized users, regardless of geographic location) varies by size of organization and ranges from \$993–\$1445 for US organizations, and \$1073–\$1526 for international organizations (air delivery); multiple campuses not permitted without special arrangement. Details of the tiered pricing system at https://subscriptionoffice.com/pages/apha-landing-page. To order, write apha.subscriptions@apha.org.

Online-only subscriptions: Institutional price for one institution and its authorized users (regardless of geographic location) is \$878–\$1307. To order, write apha.subscriptions@apha.org. For academic consortia or multisite corporate subscriptions, contact apha.subscriptions@apha.org.

Print-only subscriptions: Institutional price is US \$701, \$782 international.

Back print issues: A limited number of print issues are for sale. Single copies are US \$49, \$55 international (air delivery). Shipping included; prepay only. To order, write apha.subscriptions@apha.org.

Reprints: For prices and ordering information on 50 or more reprints, check the Reprints section at www.ajph.org. To order smaller quantities of reprints (rush delivery), use the "Purchase Article" link on the article site itself.

Electronic access: Online articles more than 10 years old are available free for personal use at www.ajph.org. Recent articles are available through pay-per-view: single PDF article for \$24, single issue access for 24 hours for \$33, or entire site access for 24 hours for \$38.

Postal information: Periodicals postage paid at Washington, DC, and additional mailing offices. Postmaster: Send address changes to American Journal of Public Health, 800 I St NW, Washington, DC 20001-3710.

Address changes: Send to AJPH, Membership Department (members) or AJPH Subscriptions (subscribers), APHA, 800 I St NW, Washington, DC 20001-3710. Or write to membership.mail@apha. org (members) or apha.subscriptions@apha.org (subscribers).

Advertising: For pricing and other information, see www.ajph.org. Please write to ashell.alston@apha.org or call (202) 777-2470 for other advertising opportunities. Ask about special exhibit packages and sponsorships. Acceptance of advertising by the *Journal* does not imply endorsement of products.

Indexes: Publications that index or abstract articles from *AJPH* include the following: Ageline, Assia (Applied Social Science Index and Abstracts), Biological Abstracts, Chemical Abstracts, CINAHL, Criminal Justice Abstracts, EMBASE, EMCare, Environmental Abstracts, e-psyche, ERIC, ETOH (Alcohol and Alcohol Problems Science Database), Excerpta Medica, Food Science and Technology, General Science Index, Grateful Med, Hospital Literature Index, Human Resources Abstracts, International Pharmaceutical Abstracts (IPA), Medline, Physical Education Index, Pollution Abstracts, Psychological Abstracts, PsychINFO, Safety Science Abstracts, Sage Family Studies Abstracts, Sage Human Resources Abstracts, Science Citation Index, SCOPUS, SIIC Data Bases, Social Work Research and Abstracts, and Statistical Reference Index (SRI)/LexisNexis.

AJPH

A PUBLICATION OF THE
AMERICAN PUBLIC HEALTH ASSOCIATION

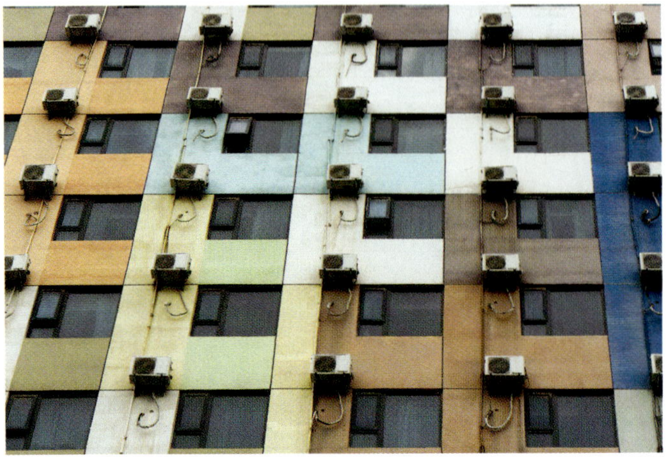

COVER: Indoor air quality and ventilation have long been a topic within public health. From the Roman architects of the first century BC to contemporary engineers working to design spaces that help combat COVID-19, clean air has often been considered a cost-effective and non-intrusive way to improve public health. But these clean air strategies have consistently lacked, and even ignored, the broader context of disparities within environmental, social, and economic realities. This issue of *AJPH* examines the notion of air quality as a public good as well as the central question: who is responsible for health?

Cover concept and selection by Aleisha Kropf. Photo by Jiojio/Getty Images. Printed with permission.

APHA
AMERICAN PUBLIC HEALTH ASSOCIATION
For science. For action. For health.

Promoting public health research, policy, practice, and education is the *AJPH* mission. As we widen our scope to embrace global issues, we also sharpen our focus to support the needs of public health practitioners. We invite contributions of original unpublished research, opinion and commentary, and letters to the editor.

The *Journal* is printed on acid-free recycled paper.

OPEN ACCESS ONLINE ONLY PODCAST DATA SUPPLEMENT AVAILABLE

EDITOR'S CHOICE

757 The US Presidential Election of 2024 Is a Public Health Emergency
A. Morabia

BOOKS & MEDIA

760 A Fresh Historical Light on the Political Economy of US Health Care Policy
L. D. Brown

OPINIONS, IDEAS, & PRACTICE

EDITORIALS

763 A Multiprong Approach to Curb Underage Drinking: Addressing a Centuries-Old Practice in China
L. Fang

766 Minimum Age Firearm Purchase Laws, by Themselves, Don't Prevent Youth Suicide
S. C. Peck

769 School-Based Health Centers Are a Critical Component of Health Care for Children: A Public Health of Consequence, August 2024
F. Kapadia

PERSPECTIVES

772 A Call for Measuring Partisanship in US Public Health Research
J. Pacheco, S. E. Gollust, T. Callaghan, and M. Motta

777 Recommendations and Implementation Considerations for the Routine Collection of Sexual Orientation and Gender Identity Data in Research and Practice
I. Tamí-Maury and T. J. Millett

782 US Maternal Mortality Solutions Must Include Addressing Intimate Partner Violence
M. P. DeMarco, J. D. Cohn, J. Dubois, T. Lapp, M. L. Donze, M. Nyachogo, and P. F. Cronholm

NOTES FROM THE FIELD

785 Rapid Response to the Legalization of Fentanyl Test Strips in Alabama: An Academic–Community Partnership
C. G. McCollum, G. Ventrelli, K. W. Gagnon, A. Loftis, A. Famurewa, C. Wimberly, and E. Eaton

789 Engaging School Champions in the Implementation of a Research Study in Historically Marginalized School Communities
T. Kenworthy LaMarca, M. Campez-Pardo, K. C. Sauvigné, G. Guevara, R. M. Fleurime, and E. R. Pulgaron

INDOOR AIR QUALITY & PUBLIC HEALTH

794 Business, Ventilation, and Health—Can We Have Them All?
M. A. Kiechle

796 The "Best of All Breathing"?
C. Hamlin

RESEARCH & ANALYSIS

INDOOR AIR QUALITY & PUBLIC HEALTH

798 Ventilation and Public Health: A Fraught History
E. LaFay and P. Sampson

HEALTH MONITORING

805 Examining the Impact of Minimum Handgun Purchase Age and Background Check Legislation on Young Adult Suicide in the United States, 1991–2020
E. E. Fridel, G. M. Zimmerman, and S. R. Arrigo

OPEN-THEMED RESEARCH

814 Alcohol Advertising Exposure and Drinking Habits Among Chinese Adolescents in 2021: A National Survey
N. Ji, Q. Xu, X. Zeng, S. Casswell, Y. Bai, and S. Liu

824 "The Hotel of 10,000 Stars": The Impact of Social-Structural Determinants of Health Among Im/migrant Shrimpers in the Gulf of Mexico
S. Guillot-Wright, L. Davis, L. Truong, H. Castañeda, and A. Rodriguez

833 Preexposure Prophylaxis (PrEP) for HIV Prevention at Outpatient Substance Use Treatment Facilities, United States, 2021
S. R. Bunting, N. Vidyasagar, A. P. Wilson, and A. Hazra

BACKMATTER

ERRATA

838 Erratum In: "Rapid Community Translation in the Colorado CEAL (CO-CEAL) Program: Transcreating Messaging to Promote COVID-19 Vaccination"

839 Erratum In: "Retention of Community Health Workers in the Public Health Workforce: Public Health Workforce Interests and Needs Survey, 2017 and 2021"

OTHER DEPARTMENTS

840 Subscription Form

The US Presidential Election of 2024 Is a Public Health Emergency

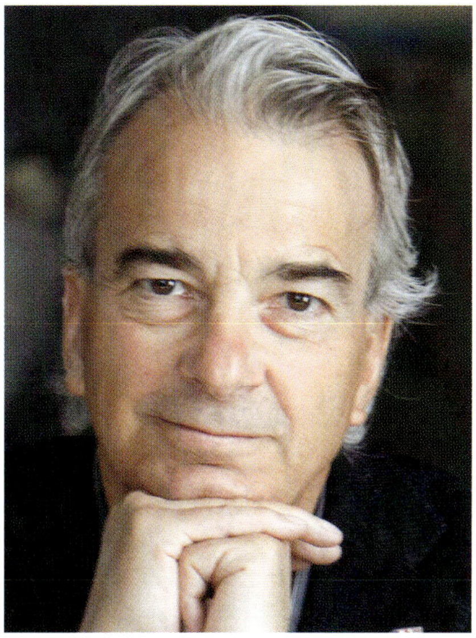

Alfredo Morabia, MD, PhD
Editor-in-Chief, *AJPH*

AJPH has relentlessly provided evidence indicating the dire public health consequences of weakening democracy and the lack of fair representation in bodies that decide how a population protects itself from all types of deleterious health determinants. A recent editorial on the Web site of the American Civil Liberties Union (ACLU), representing 6.5 million supporters, should be read as an alarming call for public health because the authoritarian plans proposed by the former president and current presidential candidate are serious:

> He has made clear he intends to deploy the military to crush protests; activate state national guards to deport millions of immigrants; build on his legacy of gutting reproductive freedoms by implementing a nationwide abortion ban; create a police state in which anyone who he views as an "enemy" is surveilled and our law enforcement are further empowered to use lethal force; and undermine the integrity of our elections. (https://bit.ly/3V7BPBq)

The ACLU describes itself as a nonpartisan organization whose primary mission is to defend and preserve the individual rights and liberties guaranteed by the Constitution and laws of the United States. In several instances, the ACLU has supported former President Trump and filed amicus briefs on his behalf against certain plaintiffs.

In the quote above, the ACLU expresses severe concerns that, depending on the outcome of the election in November 2024, the next administration could behave in a fascistic manner. This echoes the denunciation of the "fascist threat" in the April 2021 issue of *AJPH*. We wrote then that "Whether there is a serious fascist threat in the United States is debatable" (https://bit.ly/3V68JCu). Debatable? Not anymore. Our warning was largely confirmed by the bipartisan committee established by the US House of Representatives, formally known as the "Select Committee to Investigate the January 6th Attack on the United States Capitol." The call to action by the ACLU also

Continued on page e2...

HISTORY CORNER

34 YEARS AGO

Sick Building Syndrome

Indoor air quality concerns are not limited to the discomfort complaints of sick building syndrome. Building-related illnesses, distinguished by objective findings underlying pathologic diagnoses, include hypersensitivity, pneumonitis, asthma, and infections such as legionellosis. These are frequently related to humidification systems or other components of temperature control. Building-related illness occurs in settings which also have high complaint rates of symptoms consistent with sick building syndrome. Whether this coincidence points to a common source is unclear. Building and ventilation design characteristics may have major public health implications for transmission of communicable disease as well. Investigators in Switzerland found increased absenteeism for respiratory illness in a fully air conditioned building, in comparison to a naturally ventilated building with a similar population. A US Army study showed a 51 percent increase in febrile acute respiratory disease in basic trainees at four army centers living in energy-efficient army barracks in comparison to trainees living in old "leaky" barracks. . . . The scientific underpinnings for solving indoor air quality complaints will only be established by systematic epidemiologic work in conjunction with ventilation engineering and industrial hygiene assessment.

From *AJPH*, October 1990, pp. 1172–1173

converges on the same conclusion: the fascist threat is real. All supporters of the former president may not be fascist, but the far-right ideology, the militarization of the police, the violent suppression of opposition, the massive deportation, the beliefs in White supremacy, and the strongman and authoritarian demeanor are undoubtedly fascist traits. These intentions are ostentatiously placed before the voters this fall. For more details, refer to the *AJPH* article, "The Fascist Threat" (https://bit.ly/3V68JCu).

We are still a few months away from the elections. The term "fight back" used by the ACLU is inappropriate. It is still possible to prevent the announced disaster, but the clock is ticking. This is a call to action for all of us, not only as citizens but as public health professionals. The regime promised by the former president may result in harmful policies from which, because of the infringements on people's liberties mentioned by the ACLU, there may be no democratic or legal recourse. Here are some examples.

DEPORTING MILLIONS OF IMMIGRANTS

The consequences of massive deportation would surpass anything we have yet seen in the United States. However, we know that even less extreme measures, such as making it more difficult for immigrants to obtain visas or green cards (i.e., the public charge rule), have visible public health consequences. In 2019, the administration threatened to expand the criteria for determining public charge to include beneficiaries of Medicaid, the Supplemental Nutrition Assistance Program (SNAP), and housing assistance. These threats produced potentially chilling effects, reducing the participation of immigrant households in federal food and nutrition assistance programs in states with more generous policies toward immigrants. In New York state, this led to delayed Medicaid enrollment for pregnant women and lowered birth weights. For more details, refer to the December 2022 issue of *AJPH* (https://bit.ly/3R9JygW).

GUTTING REPRODUCTIVE FREEDOMS

The Supreme Court's *Dobbs* decision overturning *Roe v Wade*, discussed in the September 2022 issue of *AJPH*, opened the door to extreme right-wing attacks on reproductive rights. The immediate consequences have included tens of thousands of people being turned away from receiving abortion services in their own states, leading to delays and forcing individuals to seek abortion care later in pregnancy, with some persons even being denied care during medical emergencies. Public frustration against this decision has been palpable in some elections, as many people consider resorting to abortion at some point, with about one in four women of reproductive age undergoing an abortion during their lifetime. However, the situation could deteriorate further if Congress decides to forbid abortion entirely. For more details, refer to these *AJPH* articles on the consequences of the *Dobbs* decision (https://bit.ly/4e5E7JT), the impact on abortion services (https://bit.ly/3Rb2CM2), abortion statistics (https://bit.ly/3VmsxCP), and lifetime prevalence of abortion (https://bit.ly/3VmsxCP).

Continued on page e3...

HISTORY CORNER

81 YEARS AGO

Defense Ventilation and Air Conditioning Problems

Ventilation and air conditioning are contributing an important part in production for national defense. The necessity for uninterrupted production under conditions of blackout has led to the design of windowless "blackout plants" for airplane factories, munition plants, and for other key defense industries. These plants are huge single-story buildings with few or no interior partitions. Raw materials go in at one end and finished products come out at the other. Except in cold weather, much artificial cooling is required to remove excessive heat from furnaces, machinery, and solar radiation. Aside from human comfort requirements, temperature control is essential to insure precision of finished parts for airplanes, tanks, instruments, etc. . . . An undesirable feature in the design of some blackout plants is the lack of segregation of clean from the toxic process. Air pollution may be particularly aggravated in warm weather when the outside air supply is normally reduced to about one air change per hour in the interest of economy. For small workshops and factories that are ventilated by natural methods, several types of blackout ventilators have been developed which obscure the outward passage of light without obstructing air flow too much.

From *AJPH*, July 1943, pp. 859–860

UNDERMINING THE INTEGRITY OF ELECTIONS

Making sure that voting is accessible to all eligible citizens is an element of fair elections. The US Voting Rights Act of 1965, which removed many obstacles to voting, led to pronounced reductions in infant deaths for Black Americans, which exceeded reductions among White Americans. This highlights the powerful public health impact of voting rights. However, the Supreme Court's *Shelby County v Holder* decision in 2013 removed the requirement for states with a history of discrimination to obtain federal approval (i.e., "preclearance") before changing voting policies. Since then, 29 states have passed 94 restrictive voting laws, with 11 of those states previously covered by the preclearance mandate. Voting rights could be undermined further by an administration infiltrated by White supremacists. For more details, refer to the *AJPH* article "1965 US Voting Rights Act Impact on Black and Black Versus White Infant Death Rates in Jim Crow States" (https://bit.ly/4c1plfP) and the March 2024 issue of *AJPH* (https://bit.ly/457PNHR).

COMMON GROUND

There are many more domains in which a victory by chauvinist, racist, religiously fanatic, and xenophobic far-right forces would have disastrous public health consequences. These ideologies focus on excluding and eventually destroying subgroups of the population, sometimes through industrial or warfare genocides. Such ideologies are incompatible with any form of public health.

Effective public health is inherently inclusive. The late David Sundwall, a Republican state health officer from Utah, wrote in *AJPH*:

> I call upon everyone to respect each other, to not demonize the detractors of public health, and—for those who are resistant to government recommendations—to recognize the benefits to all that will result from containment over time. And I call upon my colleagues in public health to demonstrate some humility, to acknowledge that broad-scale lockdowns of entire communities, school closures, and mandates have not proven as effective as hoped, and have been very costly, both economically and on our emotional health (https://bit.ly/456lMbC).

The October 2023 issue of *AJPH*, dedicated to "Finding Common Ground for Public Health Action," featured contributions from Sundwall's former colleagues and friends. For more details, refer to the *AJPH* articles "In Defense of Public Health" (https://bit.ly/3Vqv8M9), David Sundwall's "Public Health Across the Political Spectrum for All" (https://bit.ly/456lMbC), and the October 2023 issue of *AJPH* (https://bit.ly/4e4ynA3).

Everyone in public health cares about democracy and human rights. These values are best defended when public health practitioners engage with grassroots organizations, labor unions, religious congregations, and community leaders. The time for action is now, involving all of us. The US Presidential Election of 2024 is a public health emergency. AJPH

DOI: https://doi.org/10.2105/AJPH.2024.307737

HISTORY CORNER

98 YEARS AGO

Opposing Viewpoints in the School Ventilation Controversy

The ventilation of school buildings is just one little corner of the whole ventilation problem. However, this corner has been the storm center of more controversy than any other section. . . . There were many criticisms of the mechanically ventilated classroom and the teachers were not backward in expressing their views. The rooms were hot and stuffy, draughty and dry and lacked freshness. The teachers opened the windows to cool off; the janitor ordered them shut; teachers began getting madder and madder over these repressive regulations, and the janitors got gruffer and gruffer. . . . The final stroke which caused the American Public Health Association to burst forth at its annual meeting in St. Louis last year with a stinging resolution against arbitrary state laws on school ventilation, was a serious proposal on the part of certain people in St. Louis to compel the closing of the windows in the open air schools and the treating of the air with ozone. This was the last straw. The tuberculosis association drew the line at this and the public health fraternity went definitely on record in protest against the unwarranted invasion of the ventilating engineer into the field of public health and medicine.

From *AJPH*, November 1926, pp. 1105–1106

A Fresh Historical Light on the Political Economy of US Health Care Policy

Lawrence D. Brown, PhD

ABOUT THE AUTHOR

Lawrence D. Brown is with the Mailman School of Public Health, Columbia University, NewYork, NY.

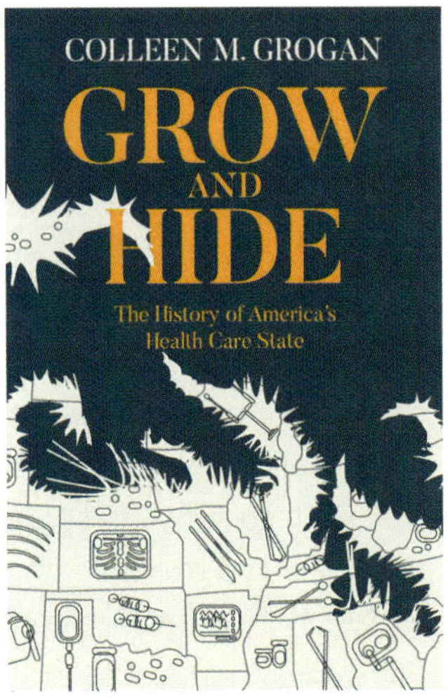

Grow and Hide: The History of America's Health Care State
By Colleen M. Grogan
Oxford, UK: Oxford University Press; 2023
448 pp.; $34.95
ISBN-13: 978-0199812233

Colleen M. Grogan's *Grow and Hide: The History of America's Health Care State* throws bright and fresh historical light on the political economy of US health care policy. The book examines the "hidden"[1] and "submerged"[2] features of US social policy and explores in extraordinary depth their sources, evolution, and outcomes in health policy.

The basic argument is that despite familiar homilies about the limited role of government in the predominantly private US health care system, the role of government—local, state, and federal—has been sizable, indeed sometimes definitive, throughout the 20th century and continues to grow ever more so in the 21st. All along, however, the growth of this public presence has been deliberately hidden: the public is assured that subnational, voluntary, and private entities run the show, not a corps of politicians. The consequences of this surreptitious strategy should worry the citizenry: fragmentation, inequities, and profiteering not only create (and thrive on) a lack of transparency and accountability but also go far toward explaining the inadequate value for money for which the US health care system is internationally notorious. The solution (proposed in a rather perfunctory five-page concluding chapter): "reveal and mobilize."

Chief among the book's virtues is the meticulous scholarship that documents the magnitude of the governmental presence in US health care policy over time and the central role of public health in that development. For more than 100 years, public health leaders have cherished a vision of an integrated, coordinated, comprehensive system of care, organized in regional institutional hierarchies led by scientific experts and protected from political patronage and perturbations. But the chance that such a model might be realized has all along fallen between slim and none, so public health leaders have exploited deficiencies and ambiguities in private medical practice to augment their own roles. For example, although firmly convinced that prevention and treatment should go hand in hand, they laid claims to a role in the latter only for patients with distasteful diseases (for instance, tuberculosis and sexually transmitted illnesses) and for patients unable to pay for care. And as the shifting boundaries of the "medically indigent" category (a conceptual evolution the book subtly traces) opened new opportunities for treatment under public auspices, public health professionals cloaked their incursions in disclaimers of any intent to "usurp" the prerogatives of private physicians and voluntary hospitals, thus seeking to advance strategically by stealth.

Grogan's account powerfully refutes the popular proposition that small government is the norm in US health care and anatomizes growth of government in this sector in exhaustive and authoritative detail. The "hide" part of the picture, however, invites contesting interpretations.

AJPH August 2024, Vol. 114, No. 8

The book pays surprisingly little attention to the centrality of "credit claiming"[3] and its in-one's-face concomitants, "advertising" and "position-taking,"[4] as political drivers of policy. The elected officials, policy entrepreneurs, and organizational leaders who promoted (for example) the National Institutes of Health, hospital construction under the Hill–Burton program, medical workforce training subsidies, maternal and child health services, Medicare, Medicaid, the National Health Service Corps, community health centers, the Children's Health Insurance Program (CHIP), and the Affordable Care Act (ACA) did not hesitate to claim credit for guiding the federal government into new territory. The "what have you done for me lately?" challenge means spotlighting leaderly "responsiveness" and innovation. Then, as the costs and complexities of such breakthroughs grew clearer, a complementary command—"Don't just sit there, do something," a species of "blame avoidance"[5]—engendered technocratic initiatives such as HMOs, Quality Improvement Organizations, Certificate of Need, planning, state (and then federal) prospective rate setting for hospitals, managed care regulation, and the Patient-Centered Outcomes Research Institute, which were far from transparent, but no one hid the government's determination to "get on the case." If these policies are instances of hiding, they would seem to be cases of "hiding in plain sight."

Grogan's argument, however, focuses less on the *political origins* of the growing reach of the public sector in health care policy than on what happens to policies as they are formulated and implemented. Her account indignantly tracks a political pattern, so powerful and pervasive as to constitute a "regime" (a term with odd overtones of agency), in which providers gain power by quietly supporting the expansion of public subsidies, diverting them to their own ends, and then publicly demonizing their governmental benefactors should they dare to demand that providers honor accountability to the public interest. Nice work if you can get it—and, in Grogan's indictment, the stakeholders get it repeatedly and with surprising ease.

But *how* do they get away with it? One familiar explanation is of course that "America's distinctive state structure" is simply too weak to marshal against private and professional interests the countervailing public power one sees in comparable Western health care systems with strong central bureaucracies and social democratic political parties.[6(pp25,19)] Arguably, this institutional timidity derives in turn from a long-standing, well-entrenched antigovernmental ethos that lends legitimacy a priori to the providers and dealmakers who denounce public interventions as statist intrusions into the proper provinces of markets, voluntary associations, and private medical practitioners. Grogan duly acknowledges the "discursive" underpinnings of Grow and Hide, but she does not much engage with cultural considerations and seems to contend that if only citizens understood how massive and deeply rooted the role of government in the health care system is in fact, they would come to embrace it, want more of it, and demand reform of the fragmentation, inequities, profiteering, and other affronts that disfigure that system. The key is to "de-bamboozle"[7(p274)] a blinkered public.

Perhaps the policy history of the US health care state is indeed best understood as a tale of deceit and deception contrived by the Grow and Hide "regime" Grogan dissects. It can also be interpreted, however, as the sum of the nation's improvised efforts to reconcile the unease of the polity toward big government with its demand that big government do big things for it. The practical results, to cite the titles of two excellent books by Brian Balogh, who elaborates on this thesis, are *A Government Out of Sight*[8] and *The Associational State*.[9] Is it really surprising that a society constitutionally pledged to separation of powers and to checks and balances should produce fragmented policies? Or that one devoted to "states' rights" (centuries-old code for racial discrimination) should tolerate, indeed encourage, inequities in health care programs? Or that a century of self-righteous propaganda expounding the alleged superiority of voluntary hospitals and insurers in supplying "accountability" to "the community," in contrast to the politics-saturated public sector, should convince citizens that they can get the health care they want without surrendering to government? Or that its reverence for the rights of private property should open doors to profiteering (led not only by the well-cloaked incursions of the private equity juggernaut Grogan adroitly brings to light but also by the for-profit health insurers, whose profits swell with every "reform"—Medicare Advantage, Medicaid managed care, Medicare Part D drug benefits, and ACA marketplace plans, for example—the system adopts? If the policy patterns Grogan deplores are viewed as costs that US politics "as usual" impose to achieve the genuine benefits the public believes health policies to confer, one wonders whether these fragmented, disparate, and profit-bloated benefits are worth these costs, or whether, as Grogan's account suggests, those costs are at once excessive and unnecessary.

Health care systems that embrace and resolve to preserve affordable universal coverage cannot dodge the challenges the US system reflexively obscures. Coverage that is, and stays, both affordable and universal requires public, system-wide rules of the policy game, binding on all stakeholders, that govern who is covered and for what, how funds are raised and expended, and how the supply side of the health care system is configured. Such systems do not entirely escape fragmentation, inequities, and profiteering, but they expect the national government to maintain policy frameworks that keep these threats in check. The United States does not grant government comparable countervailing power, not mainly because its providers insist on deceiving the polity about the magnitude of the public presence but rather because that polity declines to recognize the social benefits of affordable universal coverage under public governance and to manage the political tensons intrinsic to its preservation. The nation's implicit cost–benefit analysis is a cultural–structural product that settles for the policy outcomes Grogan astutely reviews: a mélange of generous subsidies to providers; limited, porous, and inequitable financing arrangements; simplistic images of market competition; and effete regulatory interventions. This mix departs markedly not only from the holistic apolitical utopia of the public health gurus but also from the transparent policy attainments of Western peers.

That "revelation" might dispel ingrained misperceptions and thus trigger "mobilization" for deep-reaching change may be too visionary a prospect by half. Be that as it may, *Grow and Hide* is that extreme rarity—a book that makes both a stellar addition to scholarship and an admirable contribution to democratic theory and practice. Enriched by Grogan's work, as penetrating as it is provocative, scholars of public health and public policy—and indeed open-minded citizens wherever they may be found—will be better equipped to interpret the import of the policy history it reveals and to ponder the range of political responses those revelations may call to mind. AJPH

CORRESPONDENCE

Correspondence should be sent to Lawrence D. Brown, PhD, Columbia University, Mailman School of Public Health, 722 W. 168th St, 4th Floor, New York, NY 10032 (e-mail: ldb3@cumc.columbia.edu). Reprints can be ordered at https://www.ajph.org by clicking the "Reprints" link.

PUBLICATION INFORMATION

Full Citation: Brown LD. A fresh historical light on the political economy of US health care policy. *Am J Public Health*. 2024;114(8):760–762.

Acceptance Date: May 12, 2024.

DOI: https://doi.org/10.2105/AJPH.2024.307726

CONFLICTS OF INTEREST

The author has no conflicts of interest to disclose.

REFERENCES

1. Howard C. *The Hidden Welfare State: Tax Expenditures and Social Policy in the United States*. Princeton, NJ: Princeton University Press; 1999. https://doi.org/10.1515/9781400822416
2. Mettler, Suzanne. *The Submerged State: How Invisible Government Policies Undermine American Democracy*. Chicago, IL: University of Chicago Press; 2011.
3. Fenno RF. *Congressmen in Committees: The Challenge of Congressional Governance*. New York, NY: Little, Brown; 1973.
4. Mayhew DR. *Congress: The Electoral Connection*. New Haven, CT: Yale University Press; 2004.
5. Weaver RK. The politics of blame avoidance. *J Public Policy*. 1986;6(4):371–398. https://doi.org/10.1017/S0143814X00004219
6. Skocpol T. *Social Policy in the United States: Future Possibilities in Historical Perspective*. Princeton, NJ: Princeton University Press; 1995.
7. Keynes JM. *Essays and Sketches in Biography*. New York, NY: Meridian Books; 1956.
8. Balogh B. *A Government Out of Sight: The Mystery of National Authority in Nineteenth Century America*. Cambridge, UK: Cambridge University Press; 2009. https://doi.org/10.1017/CBO9780511576324
9. Balogh B. *The Associational State: American Governance in the Twentieth Century*. Philadelphia, PA: University of Pennsylvania Press; 2015. https://doi.org/10.9783/9780812291377

A Multiprong Approach to Curb Underage Drinking: Addressing a Centuries-Old Practice in China

Lin Fang, PhD

ABOUT THE AUTHOR

Lin Fang is with the Factor-Inwentash Faculty of Social Work, University of Toronto, Toronto, ON.

See also Ji et al., p. 814.

Unlike tobacco and illicit drug use, alcohol use has garnered limited attention from policymakers and public health officials in China.[1] Epidemiological studies conducted since 1980 have revealed a consistent increase in alcohol consumption and incidence of alcohol-related issues in China, which they attribute to China's rapid economic growth and the concurrent elevation of average income levels.[1,2] Such trends are reflected in underage drinking. A meta-analysis indicates that 50.7% of Chinese youths aged 12 to 18 years have had at least one alcoholic drink in their life, and 24.3% consumed alcohol in the past month.[3] Male youths have higher prevalence rates of drinking than do female youths for all drinking practices except weekly drinking and past month drunkenness.[3]

STRENGTHENING ADVERTISING REGULATIONS

The study by Ji et al. (p. 814) in this issue of *AJPH* underscores different proalcohol advertising channels in China and advances the knowledge of the association between advertising exposure and underage drinking in China. Their findings echo the calls for tightening alcohol advertising regulations, including strengthening alcohol-related policy enforcement and regulating digital advertising, given the increasingly sophisticated marketing strategies adopted by alcohol companies.[1,2] The use of advertising that appeals to youths, coupled with "corporate social responsibility" strategies designed to enhance a company's public image by highlighting its involvement in philanthropic endeavors in China, mask the harms related to alcohol consumption and obscure the profit-making intentions behind marketing efforts.[1] As commercial advertising often associates alcohol consumption with glamour, excitement, popularity, sophistication, and social status, it is imperative to not only implement stricter regulations and policies on alcohol advertising but also orchestrate campaigns that challenge these positive portrayals and offer accurate information about the consequences of alcohol consumption and underage drinking.

REASONS FOR A HOLISTIC APPROACH

Although the study by Ji et al. centers on alcohol advertising, tackling underage drinking in China requires a holistic approach. Relying solely on interventions targeting alcohol advertising is insufficient for several reasons. First, although alcohol advertising is linked to underage drinking, results from a recent systematic review show that the evidence to conclude that alcohol marketing bans effectively reduce alcohol consumption is insufficient.[4] Although this result does not suggest that restrictions on alcohol advertising are futile, concentrating on advertising alone may not achieve the broader public health goals of preventing minors from initiating and continuing alcohol consumption.

Second, alcohol advertising reflects and reinforces broader sociocultural norms and values related to drinking. Alcohol consumption has been rooted in Chinese culture for centuries. As widely documented in folk and classic literature and poetry that continue to be revered and recited today, drinking is a communal activity that takes place within the social fabric of family, work, and other social networks[1] and is often regarded as a form of cultural engagement, aesthetic pleasure, and intellectual enrichment, which is distinguished from overindulgence and misuse.[5] Research in China also suggests that drinking is associated with affective, creative, and embodied experiences among young people.[6] A coordinated and comprehensive approach is needed to shift positive attitudes toward drinking among the public, and among young people in particular, with the aim of ultimately influencing drinking practices and behaviors.

Lastly, although China has endorsed SAFER, an initiative launched by the World Health Organization (https://www.who.int/initiatives/SAFER), with the aims of restricting alcohol availability, implementing measures to combat drunk driving, improving access to screening and treatment, enforcing restrictions on alcohol advertising and sponsorship, and enhancing taxation policies, SAFER strategies have not been fully implemented in China.[7] In addition, SAFER objectives appear comprehensive, but they lack a youth focus, potentially limiting the impact on deterring young people from drinking.

FROM A YOUTH DEVELOPMENT PERSPECTIVE

Effective strategies to curb underage drinking in China would integrate a youth development perspective that considers the etiology from multiple levels, accounts for gender differences, and understands the constant interplay between youths and their environments, such as families, school, peers, and the community, all within the broader sociocultural context. To counter the injunctive norms associated with drinking, public health campaigns that underscore the alcohol-related harms and risks should begin early through the schools and in education; these campaigns could demystify alcohol consumption and empower young people to start understanding the consequences of drinking and making informed decisions about their health and well-being. Given gender differences in drinking patterns and progression, such campaigns should integrate gender-specific messages and address gender norms associated with drinking.

In addition, because parents and caregivers play a vital role in preventing underage drinking and because strong parent–child bonding and communication can buffer the effects of peer pressure and social influences, it is important to prioritize parent education on alcohol, support parents in improving their attitudes toward responsible drinking, foster parental monitoring, and promote effective parent–child communication on alcohol consumption. These efforts at the family level can be particularly relevant to males, as positive parenting is associated with reduced drinking among younger Chinese adolescent boys.[8]

Furthermore, considering the stark provincial-level disparities in alcohol consumption in China as indicated by surveillance data,[9] it is vital to engage community stakeholders such as local authorities, health care providers, educators, community agencies, and youth organizations to assess and address local needs. This collaborative approach is essential for developing tailored strategies appropriate for the regional context, including effective regulation of outdoor advertising and local television commercials, which are prevalent proalcohol advertising methods in China, as suggested by Ji et al. Other strategies to consider include adding health warning messages to labels or advertisements to allow youths to make informed decisions, as well as specifying penalties for alcohol sales to minors and reinforcing policies and regulations related to underage drinking in China to curtail the availability of alcohol to youth.

Devising underage drinking prevention strategies in China would be incomplete without incorporating digital technology. Often referred to as the "technosystem," digital technology has become a pervasive force that transcends the traditional social structures of family, school, and community.[10] The prevalence rate of 96.8% of Internet use among Chinese adolescents in 2021 signifies a near-universal adoption of digital technology. Moreover, the rural–urban digital divide in China has diminished because of the surge in e-learning platforms during the COVID-19 pandemic.[11] Digital technology provides scalable platforms for substance use prevention in school and family settings and facilitates the integration of interactive and personalized content. The current evidence suggests that digital approaches to underage drinking are effective.[12]

Drinking is a social act ingrained in cultural practices and traditions, and commercial advertising taps into these deeply rooted cultural norms to promote drinking. Ji et al. provide valuable findings on the prevalence of exposure to alcohol advertising among adolescents in China and the association between exposure and alcohol consumption. Their study results demonstrate the need for increased scrutiny of and restrictions on proalcohol advertising targeting young people. Importantly, addressing underage drinking in China necessitates a systematic, multipronged approach that includes engaging multiple stakeholders and platforms to resocialize young people about alcohol and the consequences of alcohol use. AJPH

CORRESPONDENCE

Correspondence should be sent to Lin Fang, Associate Professor and Endowed Factor-Inwentash Chair in Children's Mental Health, University of Toronto, Factor-Inwentash Faculty of Social Work, 246 Bloor St West, Toronto, ON M5S1A1, Canada (e-mail: lin.fang@utoronto.ca). Reprints can be ordered at https://www.ajph.org by clicking the "Reprints" link.

PUBLICATION INFORMATION

Full Citation: Fang L. A multiprong approach to curb underage drinking: addressing a centuries-old practice in China. *Am J Public Health*. 2024;114(8):763–765.

Acceptance Date: May 28, 2024.

DOI: https://doi.org/10.2105/AJPH.2024.307738

ORCID iD:

Lin Fang https://orcid.org/0000-0002-7944-1882

CONFLICTS OF INTEREST

The author has no conflicts of interest to declare.

REFERENCES

1. Hu A, Jiang H, Dowling R, et al. The transition of alcohol control in China 1990–2019: impacts and recommendations. *Int J Drug Policy*. 2022;105: 103698. https://doi.org/10.1016/j.drugpo.2022.103698
2. Tang YL, Xiang XJ, Wang XY, Cubells JF, Babor TF, Hao W. Alcohol and alcohol-related harm in China: policy changes needed. *Bull World Health Organ*. 2013;91(4):270–276. https://doi.org/10.2471/BLT.12.107318
3. Zheng Y, Li J, Vergunst F. Drinking behaviors of Chinese adolescents over the past three decades: a systematic review and meta-analysis. *Prev Med*. 2023;173:107558. https://doi.org/10.1016/j.ypmed.2023.107558
4. Manthey J, Jacobsen B, Klinger S, Schulte B, Rehm J. Restricting alcohol marketing to reduce alcohol consumption: a systematic review of the empirical evidence for one of the "best buys." *Addiction*. 2024;119(5):799–811. https://doi.org/10.1111/add.16411
5. Da P. Tasting the good and the beautiful: the aestheticization of eating and drinking in traditional Chinese culture. *The Cal Poly Pomona Journal of Interdisciplinary Studies*. 2003;16:67–76.
6. Liu C, Jayne M. "At home" with alcohol: new insights into young people's domestic practices in China. *Soc Cult Geogr*. 2023;24(10):1827–1845. https://doi.org/10.1080/14649365.2022.2107231
7. Chinese Center for Disease Control and Prevention. Time to take actions to reduce the harmful use of alcohol in China. 2022. Available at: https://en.chinacdc.cn/health_topics/ncd_surveillance/202204/t20220429_258677.html. Accessed May 13, 2024.
8. Bo A, Jaccard J. Parenting as an inhibitor of gender disparities in alcohol use: the case of early adolescents in China. *BMC Public Health*. 2020;20(1):1098. https://doi.org/10.1186/s12889-020-09195-2
9. Zhao Z, Wang L, Zhang M, et al. Geographic distribution of alcohol use among Chinese adults—China, 2015. *China CDC Wkly*. 2020;2(7):98–103. https://doi.org/10.46234/ccdcw2020.029
10. Johnson GM. Internet use and child development: validation of the ecological techno-subsystem. *J Educ Technol Soc*. 2010;13(1): 176–185.
11. China Internet Network Information Center. National report on Internet use by minors, 2021. 2022. Available at: https://www.cnnic.net.cn/NMediaFile/2022/1201/MAIN1669871621762HOSKOXCEP1.pdf. Accessed May 10, 2024.
12. Hutton A, Prichard I, Whitehead D, et al. mHealth interventions to reduce alcohol use in young people: a systematic review of the literature. *Compr Child Adolesc Nurs*. 2020;43(3):171–202. https://doi.org/10.1080/24694193.2019.1616008

Minimum Age Firearm Purchase Laws, by Themselves, Don't Prevent Youth Suicide

Sarah C. Peck, JD

ABOUT THE AUTHOR

Sarah C. Peck is the director of UnitedOnGuns, a nonpartisan initiative of the Public Health Advocacy Institute, Northeastern University School of Law, Boston, MA.

See also Fridel et al., p. 805.

Suicide is the leading cause of gun deaths in the United States, accounting for 60% of them (higher in some states, such as Vermont at 88%).[1,2] This statistic may be surprising given the overwhelming focus on public mass shootings, which account for less than 1% of gun deaths.[3] Nearly 30 000 Americans die by firearm suicide each year.[4] According to the National Institute of Mental Health, suicide is the third leading cause of death for Americans aged 18 to 20 years, and the rate of youth suicide is rising.[5]

To reduce gun violence overall, and to protect vulnerable youths from suicide, elected leaders and public health officials should prioritize suicide prevention. Currently, 17 states and the District of Columbia have done that by passing minimum age legislation that prohibits young adults (ages 18–20) from purchasing handguns. Of these, eight also prohibit the sale of long guns (i.e., rifles and shotguns). One state prohibits the sale of semiautomatic rifles to purchasers younger than 21 years old.[6] In this issue of *AJPH*, Fridel et al. (p. 805) report the results of their research on the efficacy of these laws.

It would seem obvious that state minimum age laws would lower suicide rates among young adults by restricting access to firearms, the most lethal means of suicide by far. This public health approach (so-called "means restriction") has strong empirical support.[7] Most people who attempt suicide act on impulse. Restricting access to the means of suicide can save a life at a fleeting moment of crisis. One expert provided this example: "When a fence barrier was installed on the Duke Ellington Memorial Bridge [in Washington, DC], suicide deaths from the bridge were reduced by 90%—and it did not increase the rate of attempts at other bridges around [the city]."[8] Applying this model to firearms *should* reduce suicide mortality.

However, according to Fridel et al., state laws that prohibit *handgun* sales to purchasers aged younger than 21 years have only a negligible impact on the suicide rate of young adults. They offer three possible explanations. First, federal law already prohibits the sale of handguns by federally licensed firearms dealers (e.g., gun shops) to purchasers younger than 21. However, these laws do not apply to *private* sellers—for example, family and friends, and individuals selling firearms at gun shows and online. (The White House recently promulgated a new rule that may limit these private sales.)[9] Thus, state laws prohibiting the sale of handguns to young adults relate only to the *private* sale of handguns. Fewer than 22% of gun purchases are through a private seller,[10] only some of those sales are for handguns, and only a small percentage of those involve purchasers younger than 21. Thus, few young adult purchasers are affected by state age restrictions.

Second, in states that prohibit the private sale of handguns to young adults, they may still purchase long guns. This may in part explain why the rate of suicide committed with a long gun instead of a handgun is higher among the young adult population (according to the authors, the rate is 37% compared with 25% in the general population). Federal law does not prohibit the sale of long guns to purchasers younger than 21. Thus, state minimum age laws that prohibit the sale of handguns *and* long guns to young adults may be somewhat more effective than those focused only on handgun sales.

The third, and perhaps most important, reason is that 75% of the firearms used by young adults to commit suicide belonged to someone else, so the state age restriction didn't apply. Notably, over 80% of mass shootings in K-12 (kindergarten to 12th grade) schools also involved a firearm that belonged to someone else.[11] These facts highlight the importance of secure firearm storage in preventing both suicide and mass shootings committed by young adults.[12]

Importantly, the authors found that the efficacy of state minimum age laws was *significantly increased* when accompanied by a "permit-to-purchase" law. These laws are more restrictive than federal background check laws, which require a dealer to run a form completed by the purchaser through the National Instant Criminal Background Check System to search for disqualifiers, including age. In contrast, permit-to-purchase laws require a would-be purchaser to apply for a permit in person with a local or state law enforcement agency. The permitting process includes taking fingerprints and an *enhanced* state and federal background check, which may have a deterrent effect on young adults in crisis. In states with only a minimum age law, suicide rates decreased by 12%, an average of two people per state. In comparison, in states with both a minimum age law and a permit-to-purchase law, the young adult suicide rate decreased by 39% and the overall suicide incidence rate decreased by 14%, with no effect on the nonfirearm suicide rate.

Based on these results, the authors concluded that state permit-to-purchase laws represent a promising avenue for reducing young adult suicide. They noted a growing body of research finding that permit-to-purchase laws reduce both suicide and homicide, and 75% public support for these laws. As these laws vary from state to state, the authors called for more research to understand which provisions are the most effective in reducing suicide, both for young adults and the general population. For example, some states had a permit requirement for handguns only. Extending the permit requirement to long guns may increase the efficacy of these laws.

The authors also considered the effect of state background check laws (which apply to private sales) on preventing young adult suicide. They concluded that permit-to-purchase laws were more promising. Still, the authors suggested further research to examine the impact of weapon-specific minimum age and background check legislation on suicide.

Permit-to-purchase laws may not be politically feasible in some states despite their promise and popular support. Of course, youth suicide is a compelling issue to most elected officials across the political spectrum, and states do change their position on gun legislation over time. So, these laws should be considered as part of a comprehensive strategy to reduce youth suicide (and all forms of gun violence). However, their impact on young adult suicide may be small, saving as few as 300 lives per year according to the authors' statistics. Given the magnitude of the problem, government and public health officials should also focus on *nonlegislative* approaches to suicide prevention.

Perhaps the most important of these is secure firearm storage. Research shows that this "means restriction" approach reduces all forms of gun violence, including those that threaten our youths: suicide, unintentional gun deaths, and school mass shootings. Government officials, health care providers, educators, suicide prevention advocates, gun violence prevention groups, gun owners, and even artists can save lives by promoting the importance of secure firearm storage to their constituencies. AJPH

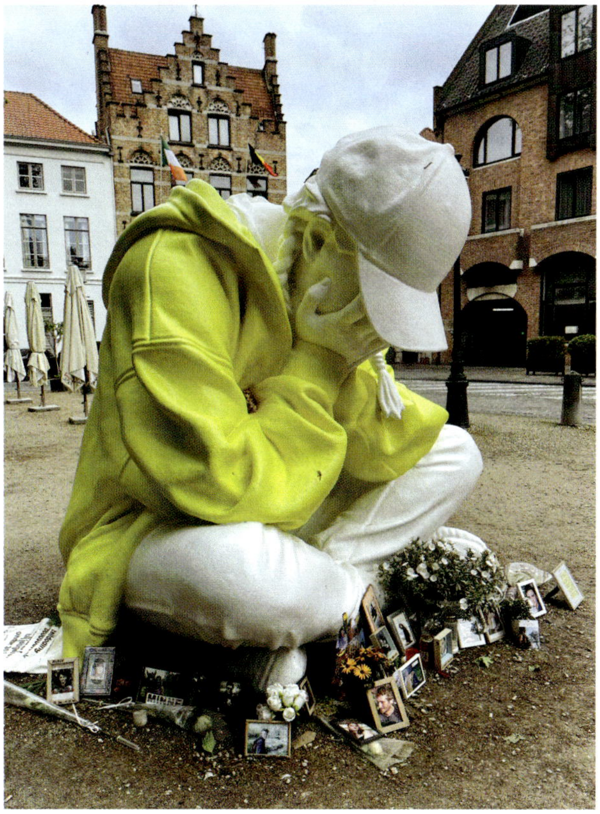

FIGURE 1— Statue of a Troubled Child in Bruges, Belgium

Note. The accompanying sign informs passersby that suicide is a leading cause of death among people younger than 30 years and provides links to a Web site with resources. Statue by SAZZA from Power of Art House. Photo by Sarah C. Peck.

CORRESPONDENCE

Correspondence should be sent to Sarah C. Peck, PO Box 335, Townshend, VT 05353 (e-mail: s.peck@phai.org). Reprints can be ordered at https://www.ajph.org by clicking the "Reprints' link.

PUBLICATION INFORMATION

Full Citation: Peck SC. Minimum age firearm purchase laws, by themselves, don't prevent youth suicide. *Am J Public Health*. 2024;114(8): 766–768.

Acceptance Date: May 24, 2024.

DOI: https://doi.org/10.2105/AJPH.2024.307734

ORCID iD:
Sarah C. Peck https://orcid.org/0009-0006-6363-6294

ACKNOWLEDGMENTS

I thank my Public Health Advocacy Institute (PHAI) colleagues Richard A. Daynard and Mark A. Gottlieb for five years of support and encouragement.

CONFLICTS OF INTEREST

The author has no conflicts of interest to report.

REFERENCES

1. Centers for Disease Control and Prevention. Deaths: final data for 2017. National Vital Statistics Report. Available at: https://www.cdc.gov/nchs/data/nvsr/nvsr68/nvsr68_09-508.pdf. Accessed May 12, 2024.
2. Educational Fund to Stop Gun Violence. Vermont gun deaths: 2019. Available at: https://efsgv.org/state/vermont. Accessed May 12, 2024.
3. Educational Fund to Stop Gun Violence. Mass shootings. Available at: https://efsgv.org/learn/type-of-gun-violence/mass-shootings. Accessed May 12, 2024.
4. Centers for Disease Control and Prevention, National Center for Health Statistics. Suicide and self-harm injury. Available at: https://www.cdc.gov/nchs/fastats/suicide.htm. Accessed May 12, 2024.
5. Centers for Disease Control and Prevention, National Center for Health Statistics. Suicide and homicide death rates among youth and young adults aged 10–24: United States, 2001–2021. Available at: https://www.cdc.gov/nchs/products/databriefs/db471.htm. Accessed May 12, 2024.
6. Giffords Law Center. Minimum age to purchase & possess. Available at: https://giffords.org/lawcenter/gun-laws/policy-areas/who-can-have-a-gun/minimum-age. Accessed May 12, 2024.
7. Substance Abuse and Mental Health Services Administration. Lethal means safety for suicide prevention. Available at: https://www.samhsa.gov/blog/lethal-means-safety-suicide-prevention. Accessed May 12, 2024.
8. Jed Foundation. I am a gun owner and suicidologist: here's what you need to know to keep young people safe. Available at: https://jedfoundation.org/i-am-a-gun-owner-and-suicidologist-heres-what-you-need-to-know-to-keep-young-people-safe. Accessed May 12, 2024.
9. The White House. Fact Sheet. Biden–Harris administration announces new action to implement bipartisan safer communities act, expanding firearm background checks to fight gun crime. Available at: https://www.whitehouse.gov/briefing-room/statements-releases/2024/04/11/fact-sheet-biden-harris-administration-announces-new-action-to-implement-bipartisan-safer-communities-act-expanding-firearm-background-checks-to-fight-gun-crime. Accessed June 3, 2024.
10. Miller M, Hepburn L, Azrael D. Firearm acquisition without background checks: results of a national survey. *Ann Intern Med.* 2017;166(4):233–239. https://doi.org/10.7326/M16-1590
11. National Institute of Justice. Public mass shootings: database amasses details of a half century of US mass shootings with firearms, generating psychosocial histories. Available at: https://nij.ojp.gov/topics/articles/public-mass-shootings-database-amasses-details-half-century-us-mass-shootings. Accessed May 12, 2024.
12. American Psychological Association. APA adopts resolution on secure firearms storage to prevent suicides. Available at: https://www.apa.org/news/press/releases/2024/02/securing-firearms-storage-prevent-suicides. Accessed May 12, 2024.

School-Based Health Centers Are a Critical Component of Health Care for Children: A Public Health of Consequence, August 2024

Farzana Kapadia, PhD, MPH

ABOUT THE AUTHOR

Farzana Kapadia is the deputy editor of the American Journal of Public Health *and professor of epidemiology at the School of Global Public Health, New York University, New York, NY.*

See also Kenworthy LaMarca et al., p. 789.

School-based health centers (SBHCs) represent an important entry point for access to timely, appropriate, and necessary preventative and treatment-specific health care for children. The presence of health services within schools enhances equitable access, reduces stigma, and allows for early intervention—often the most important driver of positive health outcomes. In addition to physicians, many SBHCs include nurse practitioners, dental hygienists, physician assistants, dieticians, social workers, and mental health specialists. SBHCs serve as a safety net and are often the only source of health care services for children who are medically underserved, lack insurance, or are underinsured. Importantly, the ability to access services in school often prevents unnecessary absenteeism and increases the likelihood that children will stay on track educationally.

To understand precisely why SBHCs have become a critical component of ensuring health care access to medically underserved children, this editorial provides context on the status of health care access and quality of care for children in the United States. Next, a summary of evidence published in the *Journal* on how SBHCs provide health care access to children is presented to support the growing need for SBHCs as a means of ensuring that children in the United States receive the health care they need and deserve.

GAPS IN HEALTH INSURANCE COVERAGE FOR CHILDREN

Between 2019 and 2021, the proportion of uninsured children in the United States aged birth to 17 years declined from 5.1% to 4.2% (https://bit.ly/4aG0XVK). This decline was largely attributed to pandemic-era legislation preventing disenrollment of Medicaid and Children's Health Insurance Program (CHIP) beneficiaries by requiring states to maintain continuous enrollment during the federally declared COVID-19 public health emergency (https://bit.ly/3V8z1VL). Despite these gains, three major challenges to ensuring the health and well-being of all children in the United States persist. First, racial and ethnic as well as geographic inequities in health insurance coverage for children remain stark. A KFF analysis of 2022 American Community Survey data found that American Indian and Alaskan Native (11.9%), Native Hawaiian or Other Pacific Islander (9.6%), and Hispanic/Latino (8.1%) children aged birth to 18 years were more likely to be uninsured than their White peers (3.9%). Second, by race and ethnicity, White, Hispanic, Black, Asian, and Native Hawaiian or Other Pacific Islander children in Medicaid nonexpansion states were more likely to be uninsured than their peers in Medicaid expansion states (https://bit.ly/3US4Dxy). Third, with the end of continuous enrollment on March 31, 2023, states are struggling to renew eligibility for all Medicaid and CHIP enrollees by May 2024. This struggle signals growing concerns about the possibility of reversing the declines in insurance coverage for children (https://bit.ly/3Kf0r6b).

INEQUITIES IN HEALTH CARE FOR CHILDREN

Inequities in the quality of health care children receive persist and are heightened for minoritized children. A 2024 review of studies examining racial and ethnic inequities in the quality of health care services for children found that, compared with their White peers,

AJPH August 2024, Vol. 114, No. 8

children from minoritized backgrounds experienced poor quality of communication between health care providers and families, longer wait times and evaluation of suspected child abuse, and disparities in the diagnosis of developmental disabilities as well as in mental health diagnosis and care.[1] A 2022 KFF report found that children living in lower-income households were also more likely to have missed or delayed a preventative health care visit than those living in higher-income households (https://bit.ly/3USHqeH). Finally, for all children, mental health needs have been exacerbated by the COVID-19 pandemic. Despite these needs, a recent federal policy brief noted that older children aged 12 to 17 years received the lowest rates of preventative care for depression and suicide risk.[2]

Thus, we are at a point where the potential for significant and immediate loss of insurance coverage, coupled with ongoing inequities in the quality and timeliness of care that children receive, may undermine the health of our population's most vulnerable and underserved children. Subsequently, SBHCs may be in greater demand across the United States and play an even greater role in providing basic preventative care, mental health services, and access to community resources.

IMPACT OF SCHOOL-BASED HEALTH CENTERS

There is a strong body of literature on the effectiveness of SBHCs in providing a wide range of health care services and positively affecting health outcomes among children. As early as 2011, McNall et al. reported that children in Michigan who frequented SBHCs in their middle and high schools reported greater overall satisfaction with their health, increased engagement in physical activity, and consumption of healthier foods compared with nonusers.[3] Simmer-Beck et al. have also reported on increased access to oral health care services for low-income and uninsured school children as a result of access to federally qualified health center–sponsored school-based dental care.[4]

SBHCs have also historically played an important role in sexual and reproductive health care provision and pregnancy prevention.[5,6] For example, Dunville et al. describe a school-based intervention for Chlamydia trachomatis (CT) screening in four Detroit public high schools between 2011 and 2015. They found a decrease in CT prevalence, from 10.26% to 6.19%, and noted that given the economic decline in Detroit during this period, providing access to school-based CT testing was the only "consistent source of publicly available testing during this time."[5(p232)] In this issue of the *Journal*, Kenworthy LaMarca et al. (p. 789) remind us that the success of interventions such as that described by Dunville et al., as well as engagement in care at SBHCs overall, can be enhanced by engaging both school staff and students to partner with research teams to promote SBHC health initiatives.

CURRENT STATE OF SCHOOL-BASED HEALTH CENTERS

Across the United States, there has been a growth in the number of SBHCs over the past 30 years. In New York State alone, there were 252 approved SBHCs operating as of April 10, 2023 (https://bit.ly/4bvcUi8). The design and implementation of SBHCs are guided by tools and models to ensure appropriateness and effectiveness of SBHC services. The Centers for Disease Control and Prevention's (CDC) School Health Index (https://www.cdc.gov/healthyschools/shi/index.htm) provides interactive tools to allow schools to identify appropriate and necessary services to support health and healthy behaviors for their school population. School Health Indexes align with the CDC's Whole School, Whole Community, Whole Child to provide a comprehensive model for addressing health in schools. By centering the needs of students, the model provides a framework for understanding how families, communities, and SBHCs can collaborate to enhance both the educational and health status of children. These models are also widely applied in SBHCs serving rural communities, where services have adapted to meet the changing health care needs of these communities to include substance use prevention and treatment as well as telehealth services (https://bit.ly/3wOs6Yw).

In conclusion, SBHCs remain an integral mechanism for providing medically underserved youths across the United States with timely, appropriate, and quality physical and mental health care services. SBHCs eliminate known barriers to health care uptake—namely, transportation, time commitment, cost, and the fragmentation or lack of continuity of care.[7] In doing so, SBHCs promote the health of families and ensure that communities espouse a shared commitment to the health and well-being of children. Investments in SBHCs also represent investments in the social and economic well-being of children into adulthood—which, in turn, is an investment in the health of our future. AJPH

CORRESPONDENCE

Correspondence should be sent to Farzana Kapadia, PhD, MPH, New York University, School of Global Public Health, 708 Broadway,

Room 729, New York, NY 10003 (e-mail: farzana.kapadia@nyu.edu). Reprints can be ordered at https://www.ajph.org by clicking the "Reprints" link.

PUBLICATION INFORMATION

Full Citation: Kapadia F. School-based health centers are a critical component of health care for children: a public health of consequence, August 2024. *Am J Public Health*. 2024;114(8): 769–771.

Acceptance Date: May 24, 2024.

DOI: https://doi.org/10.2105/AJPH.2024.307736

ORCID iD:

Farzana Kapadia https://orcid.org/0000-0003-3459-767X

CONFLICTS OF INTEREST

The author has no conflicts of interest to disclose.

REFERENCES

1. Slopen N, Chang AR, Johnson TJ, et al. Racial and ethnic inequities in the quality of paediatric care in the USA: a review of quantitative evidence. *Lancet Child Adolesc Health*. 2024;8(2):147–158. https://doi.org/10.1016/S2352-4642(23)00251-1
2. Conmy AB, Peters C, De Lew N, Sommers BD. Children's health coverage trends: gains in 2020–2022 reverse previous coverage losses. Issue Brief No. HP-2023-07. Office of the Assistant Secretary for Planning and Evaluation, US Dept of Health and Human Services. March 2023. Available at: https://aspe.hhs.gov/sites/default/files/documents/77d7cc41648a371e0b5128f0dec2470e/aspe-childrens-health-coverage.pdf. Accessed May 15, 2024.
3. McNall MA, Lichty LF, Mavis B. The impact of school-based health centers on the health outcomes of middle school and high school students. *Am J Public Health*. 2010;100(9):1604–1610. https://doi.org/10.2105/AJPH.2009.183590
4. Simmer-Beck M, Wellever A, Kelly P. Using registered dental hygienists to promote a school-based approach to dental public health. *Am J Public Health*. 2017;107(S1):S56–S60. https://doi.org/10.2105/AJPH.2017.303662
5. Dunville R, Peterson A, Liddon N, Roach M, Coleman K, Dittus P. Sustained reduction in chlamydia infections following a school-based screening: Detroit, 2010–2015. *Am J Public Health*. 2018;108(2):231–233. https://doi.org/10.2105/AJPH.2017.304163
6. Denny S, Robinson E, Lawler C, et al. Association between availability and quality of health services in schools and reproductive health outcomes among students: a multilevel observational study. *Am J Public Health*. 2012;102(10):e14–e20. https://doi.org/10.2105/AJPH.2012.300775
7. Love HE, Schlitt J, Soleimanpour S, Panchal N, Behr C. Twenty years of school-based health care growth and expansion. *Health Aff (Millwood)*. 2019;38(5):755–764. https://doi.org/10.1377/hlthaff.2018.05472

A Call for Measuring Partisanship in US Public Health Research

Julianna Pacheco, PhD, Sarah E. Gollust, PhD, Timothy Callaghan, PhD, and Matthew Motta, PhD

ABOUT THE AUTHORS

Julianna Pacheco is with the Department of Political Science, University of Iowa, Iowa City. Sarah E. Gollust is with the Division of Health Policy and Management, University of Minnesota School of Public Health, Minneapolis. Timothy Callaghan and Matthew Motta are with the Department of Health Law, Policy, and Management at the Boston University School of Public Health, Boston, MA.

AJPH August 2024, Vol. 114, No. 8

An important lesson learned from COVID-19 is that partisanship matters. Democrats and Republicans differed on a host of behaviors including masking, vaccination, and social distancing.[1,2] In fact, the impact of partisanship on COVID-19–related attitudes and behaviors overwhelmed other widely studied explanations including education and income.[1] This led to differential infection and mortality rates across communities. In one study, majority-Republican counties experienced 72.9 additional deaths per 100 000 people relative to majority-Democrat counties.[3] These partisan divides surprised many in the medical and public health communities.

In this commentary, we make the case that US-based public health researchers—including researchers designing survey-based studies and agencies that conduct health surveys for surveillance and research purposes—should ask questions about partisanship as part of their demographic data collection. Zero of the 69 surveys conducted and publicly available from the Centers for Disease Control and Prevention, including vital surveys like the Behavioral Risk Factor Surveillance System, the National Health Interview Survey, and the National Health and Nutrition Examination Survey, include a measure of partisanship. (This finding is derived from automated search procedures, which we make available in the material available as a supplement to the online version of this article at https://ajph.org.)

Not accounting for the role of partisanship on health might lead to ineffective policy and health promotion interventions if partisan differences are not properly targeted. In some cases, our interventions could even lead to resistance among those needing care, potentially exacerbating health inequalities if certain target groups are motivated by partisan dispositions to reject them—a possibility that has empirical evidence.[4,5] In short, the exclusion of partisanship from public health surveys limits our understanding of scientific phenomena and our capacity for advancing population health and health equity.

WHAT IS PARTISANSHIP?

It is important to begin by defining partisanship. (We use the terms partisanship, party identification, and partisan identity interchangeably; ideology is conceptually different.) There is an emerging view in the political science literature that social groups theory explains partisan ties. According to this view, party attachments are formed based on enduring group loyalties and social identities that are formed early in the life course alongside other identities, like race and gender.[6] Parents are critical in this socialization process, teaching children about which groups "belong" to each party and how their "self-conceptions" fit into those groups.[7] Parents are not the only source of partisan learning; political information may also come from sources outside the home, such as schools, churches, peers, or political campaigns.

Partisanship is distinct from behaviors that some may deem private or sensitive (e.g., party registration, vote choice), other political orientations (e.g., political ideology, beliefs about core American values), support for political candidates (e.g., Trump vs. Biden), or policy attitudes (e.g., support for the Affordable Care Act). All of these factors are correlated with one another (e.g., a Republican tends to vote for Republican candidates), but partisan identity is a distinct concept that is captured by this single construct.

The fact that partisanship serves as a form of social identity combined with the increasingly polarized political environment means that, for many Americans, partisanship is central to their understanding of their worldview and sense of self.[8] Partisanship also helps individuals navigate their social worlds. Democrats and Republicans increasingly dislike candidates of the opposing party and hold negative stereotypes of opposing partisans,[9] a phenomenon known as affective polarization. Some even suggest that Americans' deep level of affective polarization rivals longstanding race-based animosity.[10]

It is perhaps unsurprising, then, that partisanship shapes a wide range of attitudes and behaviors in domains that are not expressly connected to electoral politics. Health is one of those domains. There is a long literature demonstrating that Republicans and Democrats have different health policy attitudes (e.g., toward government safety net programs like Medicaid or the Affordable Care Act).[11] Critically, however, they also differ on a host of health outcomes and behaviors.

PARTISAN DETERMINANTS OF PUBLIC HEALTH

Most research linking partisanship to public health is conducted at the aggregate level, no doubt because partisanship questions are rarely asked in individual health surveys. While this brief commentary is not meant to be a comprehensive review of the literature, the existing—albeit limited—research suggests an association between partisanship and health, even long before the onset of COVID-19. For instance, older data from the General Social Survey (from 2008 and before) showed that Republicans self-reported better health[12] and experienced lower mortality rates compared with Democrats.[13] In addition, adolescents who reported being healthy were more likely to identify with the Republican party in young adulthood.[14] Other research shows that depression scores have increased in recent years among adolescents who identify as female and liberal.[15] We stress that research describing partisan differences in health outcomes across the life course is spotty, and more research is needed to document these patterns as well as to understand changes in the relationship between partisanship and health over time. Documenting partisan differences may also give researchers a sense of where more work needs to be done to design and target interventions.

Identifying the existence of partisan differences in health outcomes is a necessary precondition for exploring the mechanisms that explain those differences. One possibility is that health is partially explained by partisan variations in health behaviors. One 2018 study suggested that Democrats have higher odds of cigarette smoking and excessive drinking compared with Republicans, while Republicans report more unhealthy eating habits compared with Democrats.[16] Republicans are also less likely to intend to vaccinate, not only against COVID-19[17] but also against influenza[4] and human papillomavirus,[18] and when presented with hypothetical vaccines that prevent cancer or Alzheimer's disease.[19]

Partisan differences in health outcomes may also be driven, at least in part, by the different channels that Democrats and Republicans use to access health information.[20] This can create partisan gulfs in perspectives and, in turn, lead to differences in health attitudes, endorsement of mis- or disinformation, and the over- or underestimation of health risks based on partisanship.[21,22] There are likely other mechanisms that explain partisan differences in health outcomes, but such mechanisms cannot be explored without readily available data on partisanship.

CONSEQUENCES OF THE STATUS QUO

Besides not being able to document or explain partisan differences in health, not including partisan identity is problematic for at least three additional reasons.

First is the problem of unobserved heterogeneity. As documented in the preceding section, partisan identity plays a powerful role in shaping Americans' health attitudes and behaviors. Failing to account for partisanship may imply that existing insights about the social, psychological, or demographic determinants of health are either improperly estimated (i.e., as a consequence of failing to account for the competing influences of partisanship) or fail to identify important partisan differences in health attitudes and behavior (both in observational studies and the estimation of experimental treatment effects). Partisanship's omission additionally removes the opportunity to understand how it may moderate other well-studied social determinants of health including education, income, and other sociodemographic characteristics.

Second is the problem of observational equivalence—that is, our inability to detect differences ("equivalence") in health attitudes and behaviors because of incomplete data collection ("nonobservation") of the ways they might differ. A lack of partisan identity questions in widely used public health surveys may present a lost opportunity for researchers to both detect and bridge political divides in Americans' acceptance of medical or public health interventions. For example, clinicians may tailor the conversations they have or treatment plans they recommend to reflect the differing health attitudes and behaviors of the varying patient subpopulations that they serve on the basis of age, gender identity, racial identity, or other demographics. Documenting partisan health asymmetries may allow researchers to provide evidence-based recommendations to expand clinicians' responsiveness to not just social but political differences as well.

More generally, while in the preceding section we documented several differences in health attributable to partisanship, partisan identity may be influencing health attitudes and behaviors in a wide range of applications that are yet to be explored. The existence of partisan asymmetries in unexplored areas presents an opportunity for health communicators to design strategic communication messages that aim to boost acceptance of recommended behaviors in communities that may be most likely to reject them. Failure to detect these potential partisan asymmetries may imply that health communicators are missing the opportunity to take action to address partisan divides on health behaviors and outcomes. At the same time, health care professionals may not fully understand the factors that have an impact on their patients' attitudes, beliefs, and follow-through with recommendations.

Third is the problem of potentially fallacious ecological inference. Many researchers have studied the relationship between party registration, voting behavior, and health attitudes or behaviors in the aggregate. This research has yielded important insights about the correlation between, for example, support for former President Trump and COVID-19 vaccine refusal at the community level[23] or the relationship between voting for Republicans and opioid use.[24] Still, while both health behaviors (like vaccine uptake or substance use) and partisan preferences can be "aggregated up" to different geographic levels, health decision-making is ultimately an individual-level phenomenon. Ecological studies can lead to incorrect assumptions about causal mechanisms underlying relationships observed in the aggregate.[25,26] The assumption that aggregated data can stand in for the effect of individuals' partisan identity on their health attitudes and behavior is precisely that: an assumption.

THE PATH FORWARD

We recommend that public health researchers designing their own survey-based studies and agencies fielding national or state-level surveys consider including partisanship in their research. We include agencies running surveillance surveys in our recommendation even if the agencies themselves do not report findings by partisanship, as these secondary data (such as the National Health Interview Survey) are essential for researchers to use in answering important public health research questions.

Partisanship is best captured via a standard seven-point "branched" survey question that measures both the directionality and strength of Americans' partisan attachments.[27] The branched administration format breaks up this (potentially) challenging task into two more manageable pieces by first asking respondents to report whether they self-identify with a party label (i.e., as a Democrat, Republican, or Independent). It then branches to ask Democrats and Republicans whether they consider themselves to be strong or weak partisans and asks Independents whether they "lean" toward the Democratic or Republican party.

The resulting seven-point scale provides a sense of whether Americans identify as strong, weak, or "leaning" partisans, with Democratic identification on one pole and Republican identification on the other. This approach has the major benefit of being both psychometrically validated[27] and—for benchmarking purposes—has been routinely administered in the nationally representative American National Election Study since 1952. If concerned about either the financial cost or respondent burden of including two additional questions on a health survey, researchers can simply ask the first part of the partisanship question, which ignores partisan strength and just focuses on the party of one's identification.

To be sure, critics may argue that asking about partisanship is inappropriate for seemingly "objective" scientific researchers or that government-funded data collection efforts should avoid the appearance of engaging in partisan politics by directly asking respondents about their political leanings. Furthermore, some may worry that asking about partisanship could introduce response biases for other questions.

On the latter issue, past survey methodological research finds that asking questions about partisanship biases neither survey sample composition (i.e., who participates in surveys) nor how respondents answer questions about their health.[28] Furthermore, national surveys like the General Social Survey and the American National Election Study, which receive federal funding, routinely ask questions about partisanship. Moreover, when partisanship is asked at the end of a survey, there is limited concern that the previous substantive questions would or could be affected by its inclusion. Regardless, we see an opportunity for researchers to contribute to this discussion by doing their own survey experiments, supported by measurement best practices.[29] They can, for example, vary the placement and wording of partisanship questions to better understand how asking questions about party identification influences self-reported health behaviors and outcomes. Pilot studies to assess the feasibility of including partisanship on health surveys may be especially beneficial. Researchers might also explore if social desirability bias influences measures of partisan identification, although the branched question format helps identify individuals who mask their party affiliation by indicating they are Independents, but actually "lean" toward one party.

On the former issue, we suggest that the benefits to be gained from the inclusion of partisanship in surveys outweigh the potential concerns of researchers and survey administrators. Of course, any legal concerns or funding restrictions should be carefully considered. We recognize, for example, that government agencies, entities receiving government funding, or those hoping to maintain nonprofit status must remain strictly nonpartisan. From our perspective, asking about partisanship status is nonpartisan (as it does not imply an allegiance with a particular party or platform) and essential—helping to ensure that we reach accurate conclusions about the factors contributing to US health outcomes. With that said, these issues must be worked through within governmental and nonprofit entities, with changes in policy made as appropriate.

Ultimately, the COVID-19 pandemic has taught us that not attending to political differences in acceptance of and trust in particular health interventions or in public health authority writ large has important consequences for population health. The exclusion of partisanship from most public health research could be limiting scientific advancement in the field and the health improvements that could be achieved by addressing partisanship's role in individual and public health. AJPH

CORRESPONDENCE

Correspondence should be sent to Sarah E. Gollust, Division of Health Policy and Management, University of Minnesota School of Public Health, 420 Delaware St SE, MMC 729 Mayo, Minneapolis, MN 55455 (e-mail: sgollust@umn.edu). Reprints can be ordered at https://ajph.org by clicking the "Reprints" link.

PUBLICATION INFORMATION

Full Citation: Pacheco J, Gollust SE, Callaghan T, Motta M. A call for measuring partisanship in US public health research. *Am J Public Health*. 2024;114(8):772–776.

Acceptance Date: April 5, 2024.

DOI: https://doi.org/10.2105/AJPH.2024.307691

ORCID iDs:

Julianna Pacheco https://orcid.org/0000-0002-1166-6612

Sarah E. Gollust https://orcid.org/0000-0001-6109-5953

Timothy Callaghan https://orcid.org/0000-0002-9056-9123

Matthew Motta https://orcid.org/0000-0002-2824-6833

CONTRIBUTORS

J. Pacheco led the drafting of the article. S. Gollust, T. Callaghan, and M. Motta contributed to the writing, research, and editing. All authors collaboratively developed the argument.

CONFLICTS OF INTEREST

The authors have no conflicts of interest to disclose.

REFERENCES

1. Gadarian SK, Goodman SW, Pepinsky TB. *Pandemic Politics*. Princeton, NJ: Princeton University Press; 2022.
2. Barry CL, Anderson KE, Han H, Presskreischer R, McGinty EE. Change over time in public support for social distancing, mask wearing, and contact tracing to combat the COVID-19 pandemic among US adults, April to November 2020. *Am J Public Health*. 2021;111(5):937–948. https://doi.org/10.2105/AJPH.2020.306148
3. Sehgal NJ, Yue D, Pope E, Wang RH, Roby DH. The association between COVID-19 mortality and the county-level partisan divide in the United States: study examines the association between COVID-19 mortality and county-level political party affiliation. *Health Aff (Millwood)*. 2022;41(6):853–863. https://doi.org/10.1377/hlthaff.2022.00085
4. Nyhan B, Reifler J. Does correcting myths about the flu vaccine work? An experimental evaluation of the effects of corrective information. *Vaccine*. 2015;33(3):459–464. https://doi.org/10.1016/j.vaccine.2014.11.017
5. Chockalingam V, Wu V, Berlinski N, et al. The limited effects of partisan and consensus messaging in correcting science misperceptions. *Research & Politics*. 2021;8(2):20531680211014980. https://doi.org/10.1177/20531680211014980
6. Lay JC, Holman MR, Greenlee JS, Oxley ZM, Bos AL. Partisanship on the playground: expressive party politics among children. *Polit Res Q*. 2023;76(3):1249–1264. https://doi.org/10.1177/10659129221132223
7. Lewis-Beck MS, Norpoth H, Jacoby WG, Weisberg HF. *The American Voter Revisited*. Ann Arbor, MI: University of Michigan Press; 2009.
8. Huddy L, Mason L, Aarøe L. Expressive partisanship: campaign involvement, political emotion, and partisan identity. *Am Polit Sci Rev*. 2015;109(1):1–17. https://doi.org/10.1017/S0003055414000604
9. Iyengar S, Krupenkin M. The strengthening of partisan affect. *Polit Psychol*. 2018;39(suppl 1):201–218. https://doi.org/10.1111/pops.12487
10. Iyengar S, Westwood SJ. Fear and loathing across party lines: new evidence on group polarization. *Am J Pol Sci*. 2015;59(3):690–707. https://doi.org/10.1111/ajps.12152
11. Brodie M, Hamel EC, Kirzinger A, Dijulio B. Partisanship, polling, and the Affordable Care Act. *Public Opin Q*. 2019;83(2):423–449. https://doi.org/10.1093/poq/nfz016
12. Subramanian SV, Perkins JM. Are Republicans healthier than Democrats? *Int J Epidemiol*. 2010;39(3):930–931. https://doi.org/10.1093/ije/dyp152
13. Pabayo R, Kawachi I, Muennig P. Political party affiliation, political ideology and mortality. *J Epidemiol Community Health*. 2015;69(5):423–431. https://doi.org/10.1136/jech-2014-204803
14. Pacheco J, Fletcher J. Incorporating health into studies of political behavior: evidence for turnout and partisanship. *Polit Res Q*. 2015;68(1):104–116. https://doi.org/10.1177/1065912914563548
15. Gimbrone C, Bates LM, Prins SJ, Keyes KM. The politics of depression: diverging trends in internalizing symptoms among US adolescents by political beliefs. *SSM-Ment Health*. 2022;2:100043. https://doi.org/10.1016/j.ssmmh.2021.100043
16. Kannan VD, Veazie PJ. Political orientation, political environment, and health behaviors in the United States. *Prev Med*. 2018;114:95–101. https://doi.org/10.1016/j.ypmed.2018.06.011
17. Callaghan T, Moghtaderi A, Lueck JA, et al. Correlates and disparities of intention to vaccinate against COVID-19. *Soc Sci Med*. 2021;272:113638. https://doi.org/10.1016/j.socscimed.2020.113638
18. Manganello JA, Chiang SC, Cowlin H, Kearney MD, Massey PM. HPV and COVID-19 vaccines: social media use, confidence, and intentions among parents living in different community types in the United States. *J Behav Med*. 2023;46(1-2):212–228. https://doi.org/10.1007/s10865-022-00316-3
19. Motta M. Is partisan conflict over COVID-19 vaccination eroding support for childhood vaccine

mandates? *NPJ Vaccines.* 2023;8(1):5. https://doi.org/10.1038/s41541-023-00611-3

20. Gollust SE, Gansen C, Fowler EF, Moore S, Nagler RH. Polarized perspectives on health equity: results from a nationally representative survey on US public perceptions of COVID-19 disparities in 2023. *J Health Polit Policy Law.* 2023:11066304. https://doi.org/10.1215/03616878-11066304
21. Rothwell J, Desai S. How misinformation is distorting COVID policies and behaviors. Brookings. 2020. Available at: https://www.brookings.edu/articles/how-misinformation-is-distorting-covid-policies-and-behaviors. Accessed February 8, 2024.
22. Rothwell J, Witters D. US adults' estimates of COVID-19 hospitalization risk. GALLUP. 2021. Available at: https://news.gallup.com/opinion/gallup/354938/adults-estimates-covid-hospitalization-risk.aspx. Accessed February 8, 2024.
23. Albrecht D. Vaccination, politics and COVID-19 impacts. *BMC Public Health.* 2022;22(1):96. https://doi.org/10.1186/s12889-021-12432-x
24. Goodwin JS, Kuo Y-F, Brown D, Juurlink D, Raji M. Association of chronic opioid use with presidential voting patterns in US counties in 2016. *JAMA Netw Open.* 2018;1(2):e180450. https://doi.org/10.1001/jamanetworkopen.2018.0450
25. Gollust SE, Haselswerdt J. A crisis in my community? Local-level awareness of the opioid epidemic and political consequences. *Soc Sci Med.* 2021;291:114497. https://doi.org/10.1016/j.socscimed.2021.114497
26. Woolf SH, Sabo RT, Chapman DA, Lee JH. Association between partisan affiliation of state governments and state mortality rates before and during the COVID-19 pandemic. *Milbank Q.* 2023;101(4):1191–1222. https://doi.org/10.1111/1468-0009.12672
27. Krosnick JA, Berent MK. Comparisons of party identification and policy preferences: the impact of survey question format. *Am J Pol Sci.* 1993;37(3):941–964. https://doi.org/10.2307/2111580
28. Tourangeau R, Groves RM, Redline CD. Sensitive topics and reluctant respondents: demonstrating a link between nonresponse bias and measurement error. *Public Opin Q.* 2010;74(3):413–432. https://doi.org/10.1093/poq/nfq004
29. Rosema MM, Sabrina J. Measuring party attachments with survey questionnaires. In: Oscarsson H, Holmberg S, eds. *Research Handbook on Political Partisanship.* Cheltenham, UK: Edward Elgar; 2020. https://doi.org/10.4337/9781788111997.00015

Recommendations and Implementation Considerations for the Routine Collection of Sexual Orientation and Gender Identity Data in Research and Practice

Irene Tamí-Maury, DMD, DrPH, MSc, and Thomas J. Millett, MPH

ABOUT THE AUTHORS

Irene Tamí-Maury is with the Department of Epidemiology, School of Public Health; the Center for Health Promotion and Prevention Research (CHPPR); and the Institute for Implementation Science at the University of Texas Health Science Center at Houston (UTHealth Houston). Thomas J. Millett is a PhD candidate with the Department of Health Promotion and Behavioral Sciences, CHPPR, and the Institute for Implementation Science at UTHealth Houston.

During the COVID-19 pandemic, the US Census Bureau began releasing the Household Pulse Survey to collect data on the social and economic effects of COVID-19 in the country.[1] This survey collected data on sexual orientation and gender identity (SOGI), providing valuable data to understand and address the needs of individuals who identify as sexual and gender minorities (SGMs).[2] However, the survey did not include specific SGM labels beyond the terms gay, lesbian, bisexual, and transgender, limiting its ability to fully capture the diversity of SGM experiences and identities within the United States.[1]

The absence of comprehensive SOGI information has hindered the identification of health disparities and the development of targeted interventions.[3] While some data collection efforts, such as the Household Pulse Survey, have begun to shed light on the prevalence of certain SGM identities, these initiatives often fall short of capturing the full spectrum of SOGI diversity. Because SGM identities are mobile, meaning that they have the potential to evolve across the life course, regular SOGI measurement is necessary to capture the accurate identity of a patient or research participant.[4–6] This practice will avoid misinterpretation of research findings, inadequate health care provision, and perpetuation of health disparities among SGM individuals.[3,7]

SELF-IDENTIFICATION

"Coming out" is a process in which people who identify as an SGM acknowledge and accept their own SOGI and make their identity public.[8] This process often includes four dimensions: self-identification with an SGM identity, exploration of the identity, making the identity public, and becoming comfortable and confident in the identity.[9] How and when coming out takes place is based on a number of factors, including potential violent backlash and internal and external stigma, as well as managing and navigating societal expectations.[8,9] The journey is unique to each individual.

Though it might seem that coming out is a binary state of being, the process is much more fluid. A person who identifies as an SGM is not either "in" or "out"; it is likely that there are unique levels of "outness." The process is an ongoing management of a complex identity.[8] Based on safety, acceptance, support, and myriad other factors, an individual could choose to come out early or later in life. They could also choose to disclose their identity to a defined confidant or group of confidants rather than the public at large.[8]

Coming out could change how SGM individuals are identified in a health record. For example, a person who identifies as straight could come out as gay between appointments with their primary care provider. In a research study, a person who identifies as cisgender when they are recruited into the study could come out as transgender between baseline measurements and follow-up points. Without measurement at a future appointment, the SOGIs of these individuals will be incorrectly documented.

SEXUAL ORIENTATION AND GENDER IDENTITY MOBILITY

An individual's SOGI at one point in time does not imply that the identity is

AJPH August 2024, Vol. 114, No. 8

permanent.[4,5,10] Sexuality is often fluid and can change over time.[5,11,12] Gender identity can also evolve.[12] Because SOGI data are often only collected at a single time-point, changes in identities might not get captured. This can lead to incorrect interpretation of research findings, inaccurate conclusions, and a failure to address the disparities and discrimination that these marginalized populations often face.[7]

Research participants of all age groups could self-identify differently at the end of a research study than they did at enrollment, making it imperative for SOGI data to be collected routinely and comprehensively, particularly in longitudinal studies where repeated measurements often occur over extended periods of time. Researchers must understand how intersectionality can affect health outcomes. Racial and ethnic minority individuals who self-identify as SGM face exacerbated health disparities because of the complex interplay of their identities. For instance, studies have shown that lesbian and bisexual women experience higher rates of poor mental health compared with heterosexual women. Lesbian and bisexual women who also belong to ethnic minority groups experience increased stress levels, which can be attributed to the intersection of their identities within multiple marginalized communities.[13] Without collecting SOGI information, health care providers may overlook the unique mental health needs of this demographic and fail to provide targeted support and interventions.

In health care, infrequent collection of SOGI data could lead to health complications, an increase in health disparities, and further stigmatization.[3,7] A patient could be at different risk of diseases and conditions based on their SOGI at different clinical visits, making the accurate recording of patient SOGI necessary for proper treatment and referral.[7,14,15] For example, there is evidence that transgender women who receive hormone treatment are at increased risk of breast cancer.[16] If a provider does not collect SOGI information and incorrectly identifies transgender women, it is possible that those patients do not get referred to necessary care to manage their breast cancer risk. Health care providers must be informed on SGM health issues so that they have an understanding of the need for SOGI data collection.[17]

SEXUAL AND GENDER MINORITIES IN HEALTH CARE

Previous reports have shown that lesbian women and gay men experience health disparities and barriers to accessing health care.[14] Compared with heterosexual women, lesbian and bisexual women have 1.47 times the odds of disability, 1.40 times the odds of poor mental health, 1.42 times the odds of obesity, and 1.37 times the odds for cardiovascular disease. Similarly, gay and bisexual men are at increased risk compared with heterosexual men, having 1.26 times the odds for disability, 1.38 times the odds for poor physical health, and 1.77 times the odds for poor mental health.[14]

Transgender individuals also experience health disparities.[15] When compared with cisgender individuals, transgender individuals have a higher likelihood of generalized anxiety, social anxiety, depression, psychological distress, and eating concerns as measured by the Counseling Center Assessment of Psychological Symptoms-34 scale.[15]

Health disparities are also present among SGM youths.[18,19] SGM high-school students experience more substance use, bullying, poor mental health, and suicidal ideation than their non-SGM counterparts.[19] In addition, adolescent and young adult SGM cancer survivors have been shown to have increased odds of depression and anxiety when compared with heterosexual and cisgender cancer survivors.[18]

SGMs also experience disparities in health care access and utilization.[20] There are extensive barriers to care for SGMs, including insurance coverage and provider discrimination.[20] Lack of provider knowledge on SGM health issues can also prevent SGM health care utilization.[21] Providers who do not have knowledge of SGM health can often place the burden of knowledge on the patient, creating a situation in which the patient must educate the provider on their unique health care needs.[21] Transgender participants in a qualitative study discussed having to educate their providers on transgender health issues in screening for sexually transmitted infections, noting that they were more likely to stay with a provider if they were willing to listen and learn.[21] Likewise, SGM patients who experience a situation in which a provider does not listen to their unique health care needs could be dissuaded from utilizing care in the future. SOGI-based discrimination can also be a reason for SGMs to delay treatment.[20,22] At the policy level, states can have different policies regarding gender-affirming health care, meaning that these treatments could be inadequate, biased, or not covered by insurance.[20,23] This delineation creates situations in which access to health care differs by state.[23] Implementing SOGI data collection must account for these barriers and recognize that because of them, SGM individuals might be unwilling to disclose their identities.

The collection of SOGI data at clinical visits is key for addressing health disparities and referring SGM patients to appropriate health services.[7] Patient acceptability for answering SOGI questions is high, though provider discomfort in asking SOGI questions is often cited as a reason for not collecting such data.[24,25] If SOGI data are not collected, and health care providers are thus not aware of a patient's SOGI, they may not have a full understanding of the patient's health needs. This can lead to inadequate or biased care. For instance, specific subgroups within the SGM population, such as gay men, men who have sex with men, and transgender women, face higher risk of HIV infection than the general population. It is possible that individuals identifying with these groups may choose to disclose their SOGI information because of HIV-related concerns, which could benefit significantly from open discussions with their health care provider. If a patient's SOGI information is not collected during these encounters, there is a risk that these critical conversations may be entirely overlooked. Consequently, essential preventive care, such as preexposure prophylaxis, may remain underutilized, potentially compromising the overall health and well-being of these already vulnerable groups.[3,7] A similar scenario is possible with certain types of cancers disproportionately affecting specific SGM groups, for whom early detection can be crucial for timely and effective treatment.[26,27] This includes increased risk of breast cancer for transgender women who use hormone therapy and virus-related cancers (penile and anal cancer) for gay and bisexual men.[16,26] Disclosing such critical information empowers patients to equip their health care providers with the necessary information required to deliver optimal care.[7]

Omitting SOGI data in clinical settings or health research efforts creates an invisible population of people and allows health disparities to go unaddressed.[3,7] With adequate SOGI data collection, SGM populations have pathways toward health care that can work to eliminate SGM health disparities, improving research and policy decisions that impact the overall well-being of these vulnerable groups.[7]

IMPLEMENTATION CONSIDERATIONS

It is vital to recognize the potential dangers faced by SGM individuals when discussing their identities. SGMs are 8.3 times more likely to experience violent hate crimes compared with their heterosexual and cisgender counterparts.[28] Acts of violence and victimization are strongly linked to past suicide attempts, suicide planning, and suicidal ideation within SGM groups.[29] Asking SGM individuals to disclose their SOGI can expose them to significant risk, especially when they actively conceal their identity because of perceived unsafe environments. The risk associated with SOGI disclosure must be central to any discussion concerning SOGI data collection. Researchers and health care providers bear a responsibility to understand the risks faced by SGM individuals when disclosing their SOGI. Their concern is particularly pronounced in health care settings, where revealing an individual's SOGI to a provider may inadvertently compel an SGM patient to disclose their identity to their families. In cases where families are unsupportive of SGM identities, this disclosure could potentially lead to violence, psychological and emotional abuse, or homelessness for the SGM individual. Failing to consider the potential harm associated with SOGI data collection may exacerbate health disparities and violence within SGM communities.

Multilevel approaches must be taken to implement SOGI data collection. The practice must go beyond only asking SOGI questions and move to create safe, welcoming, and inclusive environments for SGMs so that they feel comfortable providing their information. Clinical settings must include practices throughout the organization that are inclusive and affirming to SGMs. These include asking patients for their preferred names and pronouns, maintaining nongendered bathrooms, updating electronic health records to be inclusive of SGM identities, and ensuring that all providers and staff have completed SGM competency training.[3,30,31] It is important that patients are informed about why they are being asked SOGI questions at multiple appointments. Without explanation, patients could think that previous SOGI information was disregarded or incorrectly recorded. Patient-centered strategies can be used to mitigate any misunderstandings or assumptions, ensuring patients feel heard, valued, and actively engaged in their own health care.[32]

Implementation of this practice in health care settings is a commendable goal, but it is not without its inherent challenges. In addition to the need to change the culture of health care settings broadly, routine SOGI data collection requires effective education and advocacy efforts targeted at health care personnel. Not only must providers recognize the importance of SOGI data collection, but they must also believe that it warrants inclusion within their limited time appointments.[25] This is a challenge when time is a barrier for any new guideline providers are asked to implement. Previous research on SOGI data collection suggests that providers feel discomfort asking SOGI questions and largely believe that they will inadvertently offend patients.[25] Addressing this discomfort through robust cultural competency training is essential. Provider support alone is not sufficient to facilitate SOGI data collection. Though the integration of SOGI data into electronic health records systems is a critical step, it introduces new confidentiality challenges. It is possible that SGM patients may only wish to disclose their SOGI to their providers while keeping this information confidential from others. Building and maintaining trust between providers and patients is crucial to ensuring the confidentiality of this sensitive information, as revealing an individual's SOGI could potentially lead to violence and harassment.

Patient intake forms are a comfortable format for patients to input their SOGI data, which would include a nonverbal and open-ended response option.[32] This model would give patients the option to disclose their SOGI and then prompt an open discussion with their provider on relevant prevention methods for their unique identities.

Researchers must engage the SGM community in every stage of the research process, ensuring community buy-in to the work.[33] Ultimately, the societal-level policies should recognize the violence and discrimination that SGMs experience and work toward protecting the community. Policy changes require thoughtful and deliberate advocacy from people and communities across the United States.[34]

Frequency of SOGI data collection is dependent on the individual clinical appointment schedule for patients and the schedule of research projects for study participants. For example, some recommend adults aged 50 years and older see a primary care doctor every year whereas for people aged younger than 50 years visits are recommended as little as every three years.[35] Specialized care often requires more frequent appointments. In research settings, participant follow-up could vary from months to years depending on the scope and topic of the study. A good practice could be to collect SOGI data if the appointment or follow-up point occurs more than six months after the last SOGI measurement, but this would require standardization and data-sharing across organizational settings.[36] There is a need for research specifically into the implementation of SOGI data collection with measurement frequency being an area in need of evidence.

It is crucial that SOGI data collection is held to the same standards across different settings.[36] The National Institutes of Health Sexual and Gender Minority Research Office[37] and the White House Office of the Chief Statistician of the United States[38] have resources available to strengthen SOGI data collection. There is a need for stronger coordination across federal agencies in this area and implementation of their recommendations in real-world settings. A national commission for SOGI data collection would provide standards, recommendations for best practices, and guidance on the frequency and method of data collection.[32]

CONCLUSIONS

While relevant steps have been taken to emphasize the importance of collecting and analyzing SOGI data to improve health outcomes among SGM populations, it is imperative to keep moving the needle forward by insisting that scientists and clinicians implement systematic and routine SOGI data collection as a regular practice in research and health care.[7,24] This will promote the expansion of evidence that will help in the development of interventions and programs that are inclusive of the diverse needs of SGM groups.[7] AJPH

CORRESPONDENCE

Correspondence should be sent to Irene Tamí-Maury, DMD, DrPH, MSc, The University of Texas Health Science Center at Houston, School of Public Health, Department of Epidemiology, 1200 Pressler St, Suite E641, Houston, TX 77030 (e-mail: irene.tami@uth.tmc.edu). Reprints can be ordered at https://www.ajph.org by clicking the "Reprints" link.

PUBLICATION INFORMATION

Full Citation: Tamí-Maury I, Millett TJ. Recommendations and implementation considerations for the routine collection of sexual orientation and gender identity data in research and practice. *Am J Public Health*. 2024;114(8):777–781.

Acceptance Date: April 10, 2024.

DOI: https://doi.org/10.2105/AJPH.2024.307695

CONTRIBUTORS

I. Tamí-Maury conceptualized the idea and led the writing of the article. Both authors contributed to writing and editing this article.

ACKNOWLEDGMENTS

This work was supported by the National Institutes of Health, National Cancer Institute under award 1K22CA237639 to principal investigator I. Tamí-Maury.

Note. The content is solely the responsibility of the authors and does not necessarily represent the official views of the National Institutes of Health.

CONFLICTS OF INTEREST

The authors have no conflicts of interest to disclose.

REFERENCES

1. US Census Bureau. Household Pulse Survey: measuring social and economic impacts during the coronavirus pandemic. Available at: https://www.census.gov/householdpulse. Accessed January 27, 2023.
2. Human Rights Campaign Foundation. We are here: understanding the size of the LGBTQ+ community. 2021. Available at: https://hrc-prod-requests.s3-us-west-2.amazonaws.com/We-Are-Here-120821.pdf. Accessed January 27, 2023.

3. Cahill S, Makadon H. Sexual orientation and gender identity data collection in clinical settings and in electronic health records: a key to ending LGBT health disparities. *LGBT Health*. 2014;1(1): 34–41. https://doi.org/10.1089/lgbt.2013.0001
4. Rosario M, Schrimshaw EW, Hunter J, Braun L. Sexual identity development among gay, lesbian, and bisexual youths: consistency and change over time. *J Sex Res*. 2006;43(1):46–58. https://doi.org/10.1080/00224490609552298
5. Mock SE, Eibach RP. Stability and change in sexual orientation identity over a 10-year period in adulthood. *Arch Sex Behav*. 2012;41(3):641–648. https://doi.org/10.1007/s10508-011-9761-1
6. Maragh-Bass AC. The "ask" is the "answer": implementing routine documentation of sexual orientation and gender identity in health care. *Am J Public Health*. 2019;109(8):1071–1073. https://doi.org/10.2105/AJPH.2019.305192
7. Streed CG, Grasso C, Reisner SL, Mayer KH. Sexual orientation and gender identity data collection: clinical and public health importance. *Am J Public Health*. 2020;110(7):991–993. https://doi.org/10.2105/AJPH.2020.305722
8. Brumbaugh-Johnson SM, Hull KE. Coming out as transgender: navigating the social implications of a transgender identity. *J Homosex*. 2019;66(8): 1148–1177. https://doi.org/10.1080/00918369.2018.1493253
9. Rotheram-Borus MJ, Fernandez MI. Sexual orientation and developmental challenges experienced by gay and lesbian youths. *Suicide Life Threat Behav*. 1995;25(suppl 1):26–34, discussion 35–39. https://doi.org/10.1111/j.1943-278X.1995.tb00487.x
10. Ott MQ, Corliss HL, Wypij D, Rosario M, Austin SB. Stability and change in self-reported sexual orientation identity in young people: application of mobility metrics. *Arch Sex Behav*. 2011;40(3): 519–532. https://doi.org/10.1007/s10508-010-9691-3
11. Tami-Maury I, Chen B, Sumbe A, Harrell MB. Timing of ENDS uptake by sexual orientation among adolescents and young adults in urban Texas. *Nicotine Tob Res*. 2022;24(3):388–394. https://doi.org/10.1093/ntr/ntab181
12. Katz-Wise SL, Todd KP. The current state of sexual fluidity research. *Curr Opin Psychol*. 2022;48: 101497. https://doi.org/10.1016/j.copsyc.2022.101497
13. Bowleg L, Malekzadeh AN, AuBuchon KE, Ghabrial MA, Bauer GR. Rare exemplars and missed opportunities: intersectionality within current sexual and gender diversity research and scholarship in psychology. *Curr Opin Psychol*. 2023;49:101511. https://doi.org/10.1016/j.copsyc.2022.101511
14. Fredriksen-Goldsen KI, Kim HJ, Barkan SE, Muraco A, Hoy-Ellis CP. Health disparities among lesbian, gay, and bisexual older adults: results from a population-based study. *Am J Public Health*. 2013;103(10):1802–1809. https://doi.org/10.2105/AJPH.2012.301110
15. Lefevor GT, Boyd-Rogers CC, Sprague BM, Janis RA. Health disparities between genderqueer, transgender, and cisgender individuals: an extension of minority stress theory. *J Couns Psychol*. 2019;66(4):385–395. https://doi.org/10.1037/cou0000339
16. de Blok CJM, Wiepjes CM, Nota NM, et al. Breast cancer risk in transgender people receiving hormone treatment: nationwide cohort study in the Netherlands. *BMJ*. 2019;365:l1652. https://doi.org/10.1136/bmj.l1652
17. Logie CH, Lys CL, Dias L, et al. "Automatic assumption of your gender, sexuality and sexual practices is also discrimination": exploring sexual healthcare experiences and recommendations among sexually and gender diverse persons in Arctic Canada. *Health Soc Care Community*. 2019;27(5):1204–1213. https://doi.org/10.1111/hsc.12757
18. Cheung CK, Lee H, Levin NJ, et al. Disparities in cancer care among sexual and gender minority adolescent and young adult patients: a scoping review. *Cancer Med*. 2023;12(13):14674–14693. https://doi.org/10.1002/cam4.6090
19. Johns MM, Lowry R, Rasberry CN, et al. Violence victimization, substance use, and suicide risk among sexual minority high school students—United States, 2015–2017. *MMWR Morb Mortal Wkly Rep*. 2018;67(43):1211–1215. https://doi.org/10.15585/mmwr.mm6743a4
20. Hsieh N, Shuster SM. Health and health care of sexual and gender minorities. *J Health Soc Behav*. 2021;62(3):318–333. https://doi.org/10.1177/00221465211016436
21. Stewart M, Ryu H, Blaque E, et al. Cisnormativity as a structural barrier to STI testing for trans masculine, two-spirit, and non-binary people who are gay, bisexual, or have sex with men. *PLoS One*. 2022;17(11):e0277315. https://doi.org/10.1371/journal.pone.0277315
22. Macapagal K, Bhatia R, Greene GJ. Differences in healthcare access, use, and experiences within a community sample of racially diverse lesbian, gay, bisexual, transgender, and questioning emerging adults. *LGBT Health*. 2016;3(6):434–442. https://doi.org/10.1089/lgbt.2015.0124
23. Bakko M, Kattari SK. Differential access to transgender inclusive insurance and healthcare in the United States: challenges to health across the life course. *J Aging Soc Policy*. 2021;33(1):67–81. https://doi.org/10.1080/08959420.2019.1632681
24. Cahill S, Singal R, Grasso C, et al. Do ask, do tell: high levels of acceptability by patients of routine collection of sexual orientation and gender identity data in four diverse American community health centers. *PLoS One*. 2014;9(9):e107104. https://doi.org/10.1371/journal.pone.0107104
25. Quinn GP, Pratt-Chapman ML, Meersman SC, et al. Barriers and facilitators to sexual orientation and gender identity (SOGI) data collection. *J Clin Oncol*. 2021;39(15 suppl):e18520. https://doi.org/10.1200/JCO.2021.39.15_suppl.e18520
26. Cathcart-Rake EJ. Cancer in sexual and gender minority patients: are we addressing their needs? *Curr Oncol Rep*. 2018;20(11):85. https://doi.org/10.1007/s11912-018-0737-3
27. Domogauer J, Cantor T, Quinn G, Stasenko M. Disparities in cancer screenings for sexual and gender minorities. *Curr Probl Cancer*. 2022;46(5): 100858. https://doi.org/10.1016/j.currproblcancer.2022.100858
28. Flores AR, Stotzer RL, Meyer IH, Langton LL. Hate crimes against LGBT people: National Crime Victimization Survey, 2017–2019. *PLoS One*. 2022; 17(12):e0279363. https://doi.org/10.1371/journal.pone.0279363
29. Barnett AP, Molock SD, Nieves-Lugo K, Zea MC. Anti-LGBT victimization, fear of violence at school, and suicide risk among adolescents. *Psychol Sex Orientat Gend Divers*. 2019;6(1):88–95. https://doi.org/10.1037/sgd0000309
30. Kronk CA, Everhart AR, Ashley F, et al. Transgender data collection in the electronic health record: current concepts and issues. *J Am Med Inform Assoc*. 2022;29(2):271–284. https://doi.org/10.1093/jamia/ocab136
31. Mansh M, Garcia G, Lunn MR. From patients to providers: changing the culture in medicine toward sexual and gender minorities. *Acad Med*. 2015;90(5):574–580. https://doi.org/10.1097/ACM.0000000000000656
32. Haider A, Adler RR, Schneider E, et al. Assessment of patient-centered approaches to collect sexual orientation and gender identity information in the emergency department: the EQUALITY Study. *JAMA Netw Open*. 2018;1(8):e186506. https://doi.org/10.1001/jamanetworkopen.2018.6506
33. Israel BA, Schulz A, Parker E, Becker A. Community-based participatory research: policy recommendations for promoting a partnership approach in health research. *Educ Health (Abingdon)*. 2001;14(2):182–197. https://doi.org/10.1080/13576280110051055
34. Clark KD, Lunn MR, Lev EM, et al. State-level policy environments, discrimination, and victimization among sexual and gender minority people. *Int J Environ Res Public Health*. 2022;19(16):9916. https://doi.org/10.3390/ijerph19169916
35. How often should you get routine checkups at the doctor? Healthline. July 21, 2020. Available at: https://www.healthline.com/health/how-often-should-you-get-routine-checkups-at-the-doctor. Accessed June 25, 2023.
36. Cruz TM, Paine EA. Capturing patients, missing inequities: data standardization on sexual orientation and gender identity across unequal clinical contexts. *Soc Sci Med*. 2021;285:114295. https://doi.org/10.1016/j.socscimed.2021.114295
37. National Institutes of Health, Sexual and Gender Minority Research Office. Sexual and gender minority measurement and data. Division of Program Coordination, Planning, and Strategic Initiatives. Available at: https://dpcpsi.nih.gov/sgmro/measurement-and-data. Accessed February 20, 2024.
38. Office of the Chief Statistician of the United States. Recommendations on the best practices for the collection of sexual orientation and gender identity data on federal statistical surveys. Available at: https://www.whitehouse.gov/wp-content/uploads/2023/01/SOGI-Best-Practices.pdf. Accessed February 20, 2024.

US Maternal Mortality Solutions Must Include Addressing Intimate Partner Violence

Mario P. DeMarco, MD, MPH, Jennifer D. Cohn, MD, Jessica Dubois, LSW, Tony Lapp, LCSW, Melissa L. Donze, MPH, Marcella Nyachogo, LSW, and Peter F. Cronholm, MD, MSCE

ABOUT THE AUTHORS

Mario P. DeMarco, Jennifer D. Cohn, Melissa L. Donze, and Peter F. Cronholm are with the Department of Family Medicine and Community Health, University of Pennsylvania, Philadelphia. Jessica Dubois and Marcella Nyachogo are with Lutheran Settlement House, Philadelphia, PA. Tony Lapp is with Cordea, Philadelphia, PA.

AJPH August 2024, Vol. 114, No. 8

The United States is currently experiencing two intersecting health crises: unacceptably high rates of both intimate partner violence (IPV) and pregnancy-related morbidity and mortality.[1,2] IPV increases perinatally and is a leading cause of maternal mortality.[3,4] Unique to the perinatal period is the anticipated or actual presence of a child that binds partners or parents indefinitely. Separation or leaving unsafe relationships may not be possible or desired by partners; remaining together simultaneously provides an opportunity for healing and an increased risk of violence. Systematic approaches addressing violence in families and relationships are required to address US maternal health outcomes.

EFFECTS OF INTIMATE PARTNER VIOLENCE

Beyond the immediate concerns for safety, health risks—including care disengagement, mental health disorders, and poor perinatal and neonatal health outcomes—have been associated with IPV, including long-term effects for exposed newborns.[5] Moreover, through adverse childhood experiences, IPV contributes to the multigenerational impacts of violence. In our region, PhillyPRAMS (Philadelphia, PA's Pregnancy Risk Assessment Monitoring System) data[6] illustrate that 8.7% of birthing persons report experiencing IPV during the perinatal period, that there are higher rates of psychological IPV during pregnancy and higher physical IPV before pregnancy, and that IPV disproportionately affects respondents identifying as Black, those with Medicaid, and those with annual incomes less than $24 000.[6]

SCREENING

Perinatal screening for IPV is recommended by all relevant medical societies, including the American College of Obstetricians and Gynecologists, the American Academy of Family Physicians, and the US Preventive Services Task Force.[7] Historically, IPV identification in health care settings has been limited to patients experiencing harm—and not those who use harming behaviors. More commonly, responses to and interventions for the harming partner have been grounded in the criminal justice system, including arrests, mandated treatments, and protections from abuse.

Despite recommendations for perinatal IPV screening, limited provider comfort and competing demands continue to preclude IPV identification and response.[8] More than half of pregnant people experiencing physical IPV before or during pregnancy reported not being asked about relationship safety.[4] In a self-study of our practice, we found that a greater proportion of our providers identified barriers in screening for patients using harming behaviors than screening for patients experiencing IPV. Although nearly half (48%) of our providers reported that they have considered asking about harmful behaviors, less than a third (32%) had a standard approach, and only one in five reported routinely asking about the use of IPV.

A CALL TO ACTION

Perinatal health care providers and health systems must overhaul their approaches to stopping IPV and its multigenerational impact.

First, we must get past the pain points of screening. Disclosures and healing that are based in trust must be built on relationships. Continuous practice improvement, which has focused on documenting validated measures should be redirected to better connect people to resources that are embedded in practices. Practice action steps should be built across all staffing levels. Systems-level approaches that make access proximal and lower barriers to connection will improve services.

Second, as patients depend on relationships, so too must practices, through the development of collaborative relationships with direct service agencies. The complexity of relationship violence and the need for better trauma-informed care demand early integration of patient advocates and support staff best positioned to ally with patients. Direct service agencies are often open to equitable partnerships that increase access to services and can support the funding of services.[9] Often, referrals to IPV-based resources look like handing someone a card with a hotline number on it, with a suggestion that the patient reach out themselves. In these instances, both people experiencing IPV and those using IPV have noted that they are not likely to reach out because of the shame and stigma of their experiences and behaviors.[10,11] Instead, warm handoff referral mechanisms remove the burden from patients and build connection between agencies.

Third, health care providers need to develop the capacity for comfortable engagement with patients who use harming behaviors. Individuals using abuse and violence affect the current and intergenerational health of their family and themselves. Rather than rely only on criminal justice–based reactions, often triggered by a significant assault, health care providers are positioned to offer help and access to services that can support behavior change. Therapeutic approaches that provide resources to families affected by IPV in the perinatal period can support problem identification, embrace the trajectories of adverse childhood experiences leading to dysfunctional adult behaviors, challenge patriarchal entitlements through psychoeducational approaches, and broaden the skills of problem-solving, negotiation, and accountability among those who use harming behaviors.

Finally, the perinatal health care workforce needs more enhanced training to address IPV in a solution-oriented way. This includes achieving greater comfort with broaching the topic of violence with all people who use or experience harming behaviors in relationships. Through normalizing the discussion of violence, we can recalibrate the conversations patients and family members are willing to have with their health care providers and potentially alter the trajectory for individuals and families.

CONCLUSIONS

The US maternal mortality crisis is certainly multifactorial but shares common roots in the fragmentation of health care services, health disparities, and social health needs that we have noted for those who experience IPV. It is possible to integrate a standardized, low-burden, universal, practice-wide IPV screening process to connect patients experiencing and using IPV with warm handoff referral services and support that is nested in system-level partnerships. The recommendations presented here would help close gaps and avoid further fragmentation by dividing patients experiencing violence from their partners and support networks during the critical perinatal period. AJPH

CORRESPONDENCE

Correspondence should be sent to Mario P. DeMarco, MD, MPH, University of Pennsylvania, 51 N 39th St, Philadelphia, PA 19104 (e-mail: mario.demarco@pennmedicine.upenn.edu).

Reprints can be ordered at https://www.ajph.org by clicking the "Reprints" link.

PUBLICATION INFORMATION

Full Citation: DeMarco MP, Cohn JD, Dubois J, et al. US maternal mortality solutions must include addressing intimate partner violence. *Am J Public Health*. 2024;114(8):782–784.

Acceptance Date: May 3, 2024.

DOI: https://doi.org/10.2105/AJPH.2024.307732

ORCID iDs:

Jennifer D. Cohn https://orcid.org/0009-0002-9084-0531

Tony Lapp https://orcid.org/0009-0004-5758-8324

CONTRIBUTORS

M. P. DeMarco, J. D. Cohn, M. L. Donze, and P. F. Cronholm conceptualized the editorial. All authors developed, edited, and reviewed the editorial.

ACKNOWLEDGMENTS

This project was supported by the Health Resources and Services Administration (grant T34HP42132-02-01).

CONFLICTS OF INTEREST

The authors report no conflicts of interest.

REFERENCES

1. Leemis RW, Friar N, Khatiwada S, et al. The National Intimate Partner and Sexual Violence Survey: 2016/2017 report on intimate partner violence. October 2022. Available at: https://stacks.cdc.gov/view/cdc/124646. Accessed May 31, 2024.
2. Hoyert DL. Maternal mortality rates in the United States, 2021. March 16, 2023. https://doi.org/10.15620/cdc:124678. Available at: https://stacks.cdc.gov/view/cdc/124678. Accessed May 31, 2024.
3. Fu Y, Fournier K, Seguin N, et al. Interventions for intimate partner violence during the perinatal period: a scoping review protocol. *BMJ Open*. 2023;13(7):e065560. https://doi.org/10.1136/bmjopen-2022-065560
4. Kozhimannil KB, Lewis VA, Interrante JD, Chastain PL, Admon L. Screening for and experiences of intimate partner violence in the United States before, during, and after pregnancy, 2016–2019. *Am J Public Health*. 2023;113(3):297–305. https://doi.org/10.2105/AJPH.2022.307195
5. Agarwal S, Prasad R, Mantri S, et al. A comprehensive review of intimate partner violence during pregnancy and its adverse effects on maternal and fetal health. *Cureus*. 2023;15(5):e39262. https://doi.org/10.7759/cureus.39262
6. Weinbrom S, Huynh MP, Gillespie K, Montgomery K, Mehta A, Kallem S. Intimate partner violence and screening among birthing people in Philadelphia.

Available at: https://mailchi.mp/6734acb59dbe/new-chart-intimate-partner-violence-and-screening-among-birthing-people-in-philadelphia?e=d0619d7eba. Accessed August 31, 2023.

7. Moyer VA; US Preventive Services Task Force. Screening for intimate partner violence and abuse of elderly and vulnerable adults: US preventive services task force recommendation statement. *Ann Intern Med.* 2013;158(6):478–486. https://doi.org/10.7326/0003-4819-158-6-201303190-00588

8. Sprague S, Madden K, Simunovic N, et al. Barriers to screening for intimate partner violence. *Women Health.* 2012;52(6):587–605. https://doi.org/10.1080/03630242.2012.690840

9. Agonafer EP, Carson SL, Nunez V, et al. Community-based organizations' perspectives on improving health and social service integration. *BMC Public Health.* 2021;21(1):452. https://doi.org/10.1186/s12889-021-10449-w

10. Dichter ME, Ogden SN, Tuepker A, Iverson KM, True G. Survivors' input on health care-connected services for intimate partner violence. *J Womens Health (Larchmt).* 2021;30(12):1744–1750. https://doi.org/10.1089/jwh.2020.8585

11. Hashimoto N, Radcliffe P, Gilchrist G. Help-seeking behaviors for intimate partner violence perpetration by men receiving substance use treatment: a mixed-methods secondary analysis. *J Interpers Violence.* 2021;36(7-8):3142–3167. https://doi.org/10.1177/0886260518770645

Rapid Response to the Legalization of Fentanyl Test Strips in Alabama: An Academic–Community Partnership

C. Greer McCollum, MPH, Greg Ventrelli, MD, Kelly W. Gagnon, PhD, MPH, Ashley Loftis, MA, Abimbola Famurewa, MPH, Carie Wimberly, BS, and Ellen Eaton, MD, MSPH

In June 2022, Alabama legalized fentanyl test strips (FTS). In response to this new opportunity to prevent overdoses, Project Linkage, Education, and Prevention (LEAP)—an academic–community partnership providing substance use prevention services—quickly purchased FTS and started distributing them in the Birmingham area. We describe how the Addiction Prevention Coalition, a substance use education and harm reduction provider, distributed 7300 FTS in the first year of legalization via Project LEAP and discuss its efforts to decrease substance use among young people. (*Am J Public Health*. 2024;114(8):785–788. https://doi.org/10.2105/AJPH.2024.307681)

AJPH August 2024, Vol. 114, No. 8

In October 2019, the Substance Abuse and Mental Health Services Administration (SAMHSA) announced a new funding opportunity to expedite services to ethnic and racial minorities at risk for developing substance use disorders or acquiring HIV.[1] The goal of the funding was to develop prevention navigator programs to provide education on HIV, links to HIV services, and education on the risks of substance misuse.

INTERVENTION AND IMPLEMENTATION

In response to this announcement, investigators at the University of Alabama at Birmingham, along with their partners at the Addiction Prevention Coalition (APC), submitted a proposal to provide HIV and substance use prevention services to youths and young adults (YYA) aged 14 to 24 years in Jefferson County, Alabama. Funded for 2020 to 2025, Project Linkage, Education, and Prevention (LEAP) has five primary goals:

1. expand the capacity of community partners to provide substance use and HIV education,
2. promote awareness of HIV treatment as prevention,
3. increase utilization of HIV prevention services among YYA,
4. integrate a prevention navigator to increase HIV and substance use linkage and coordination services, and
5. increase retention in care among YYA with HIV and substance use disorders.

Although Project LEAP is focused on preventing both substance use harms and HIV transmission among YYA in Alabama, here we focused on its substance use and overdose prevention efforts.

Of course, the worst possible outcome of developing a substance use disorder is overdose mortality. Many evidence-based interventions exist to prevent overdose deaths, fortunately, including syringe services programs, medication for opioid use disorder, and supervised injection sites.[2] Although historically opposed to many such harm reduction measures, the Alabama state legislature passed bill SB-168 to remove fentanyl test strips (FTS) from the list of banned drug paraphernalia, which went into effect in June 2022.[3,4] As one of a relatively small handful of community organizations providing evidence-based substance use prevention services in Alabama, the APC felt obliged to capitalize on the newly legal intervention using Project LEAP funds. Although not generally considered a prevention tool, FTS are harm reduction tools that allow users to avoid overdoses and eventually attain and maintain less chaotic substance use behaviors. Being a relatively small and nimble organization, the APC quickly submitted a budget amendment request to SAMHSA to purchase FTS from the drug-checking nonprofit organization DanceSafe.[5] As a result, the APC became the first organization in Alabama to begin FTS distribution.

PLACE, TIME, AND PERSONS

As a service project, Project LEAP is engaged in a variety of activities aimed at preventing substance use as well as more broadly mitigating the harms of substance use. As of July 2023, Project LEAP has promoted addiction treatment programming through social media recruitment campaigns that have reached more than 100 000 individuals across Alabama, provided 14 community presentations on substance use and HIV prevention, and collaborated with public health and HIV service organizations at 37 community resource fairs. In addition, the Project LEAP prevention navigator provided substance use care navigation and motivational interviewing to 97 YYA who were interested in prevention navigation services, most of whom were Black (n = 55; 57%; Table 1) and were recruited from a large adolescent health clinic. In addition to employing motivational interviewing to encourage these 97 YYA to address their high-risk substance-using behaviors, such as injection drug use, the prevention navigator actively connected them to substance use treatment organizations, harm reduction services (e.g., Naloxone distribution), and other health services.

By using the academic–community partnership between the University of Alabama at Birmingham and the APC that was built with SAMHSA support, the Project LEAP team distributed 7300 FTS within one year of legalization. Importantly, they distributed 1350 by the time the local health department had cleared all administrative and funding hurdles to distributing their own FTS starting in September 2022. Besides distributing to clients participating in motivational interviewing services, the LEAP team also distributed FTS at eight large community events (e.g., resource fairs, recovery rallies) aimed at providing services to populations that are at heightened risk for substance use and overdoses, such as people experiencing homelessness and persons seeking addiction treatment.

The strips were distributed in packs of five. Each pack also came with information on how to obtain Naloxone, instructions on how to contact the APC to request more FTS, and contact information for the Never Use Alone hotline. Other supplies, such as a stir stick or testing container, were not included, as these items could potentially be considered drug paraphernalia under Alabama state law. The local health department also provided Naloxone at most of these community events. There were no requirements for receiving FTS; individuals were encouraged to take the strips if they themselves could benefit from them or if they knew

TABLE 1— Prevention Navigation Participant Demographics: Alabama, April 2021–November 2022

Characteristic	Participants, No. (%)
Race[a]	
Black	55 (56.7)
White	43 (44.3)
AI/AN	3 (3.1)
Other	0 (0.0)
Ethnicity	
Hispanic/Latinx	10 (10.3)
Not Hispanic/Latinx	86 (88.7)
No response	1 (1.0)
Gender	
Male	26 (26.8)
Female	61 (62.9)
Transgender	5 (5.2)
Not male, female, or transgender	1 (1.0)
Other	4 (4.1)
Sexual orientation	
Straight	55 (56.7)
Gay/Lesbian	7 (7.2)
Bisexual	27 (27.8)
Something else	5 (5.2)
Prefer not to say	1 (1.0)
No response	2 (2.1)
Age group, y	
14–18	69 (71.1)
19–24	28 (28.9)
Total	97 (100)

Note. AI/AN = American Indian/Alaska Native.
[a]Respondents were asked to "select all that apply" for race. Four individuals selected multiple races.

somebody who could. The prevention navigator provided step-by-step training to everybody who received FTS. Recipients also received an instruction card, which is produced by DanceSafe (Appendix A, available as a supplement to the online version of this article at http://www.ajph.org).

PURPOSE

Alabama suffers from a high and increasing rate of overdose deaths, with 30.1 deaths per 100 000 residents in 2021.[6,7] In 2022, 452 drug overdose deaths were recorded in the state's most populous county, Jefferson County, 70% of which were attributed to fentanyl.[8] In 2022, the county saw a significant year-over-year increase in Black overdose deaths (13.4%) compared with White overdose deaths (7.2%).[8] Additionally, 62 individuals younger than 30 years died of an overdose in 2022, a 12.7% increase from 2021.[8] The legalization and distribution of FTS are critical for helping the state combat these disturbing trends.

EVALUATION AND ADVERSE EFFECTS

Project LEAP's evaluation team, including an APC epidemiologist, will continue to track the distribution of FTS. This will allow the team to adjust as needed to ensure that FTS distribution events continue to focus on groups at heightened risk for fentanyl overdoses.

In the first half of 2023, the team also created a dashboard to visualize the data collected from participants enrolled in the prevention navigation portion of the project using SAMHSA's National Minority AIDS Initiative Questionnaire.[9] The dashboard indicates that Project LEAP's prevention navigation participants reflect the diversity of Alabama, with more than half of the 97 participants identifying as persons of color (Table 1). Additionally, it shows that participation in the project is generally associated with reduced substance use over time (Figure 1).

SUSTAINABILITY

To continue the momentum of Project LEAP, the APC plans to partner with the University of Alabama at Birmingham and local public health departments, with whom the organization has strong working relationships, to continue FTS distribution after the SAMHSA award concludes. By using the existing infrastructure of the University of Alabama at Birmingham, the APC, and local health departments, Project LEAP can extend FTS distribution, capitalize on additional harm reduction funds in the community, and more fully assess the outcomes of the FTS distribution activities (e.g., determining the extent of behavior change via interviews with recipients). The APC also plans to

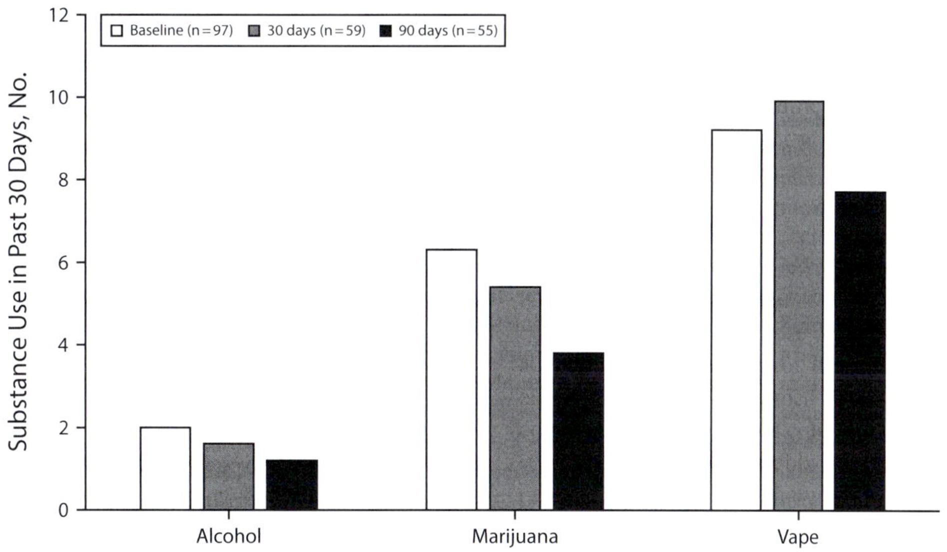

FIGURE 1— Prevention Navigation Participants' Substance Use in Past 30 Days, Self-Report: Alabama, April 2021–November 2022

Note. Because this is an ongoing intervention, not all participants have completed the 30-day follow-up or 90-day exit interview, thus the smaller sample sizes.

continue its work with treatment and harm reduction providers to ensure that those with positive FTS results can access the services they need (e.g., Naloxone distribution). The Project LEAP team anticipates funding opportunities in the near future from state and local grants, the opioid settlement, and extramural research.

PUBLIC HEALTH SIGNIFICANCE

Project LEAP demonstrates how academic–community partnerships can effectively capitalize on opportunities found in newly passed legislation, such as the legalization of FTS in Alabama, when addressing a public health crisis. A relatively inexpensive intervention, FTS are 96% to 100% effective at detecting fentanyl and allow drug users to test their supply for the extremely potent chemical before using.[10] It is recommended that persons who detect fentanyl trial a small test dose first, reduce the amount they use, use with a safer method (insufflate instead of inject), or decrease use altogether. Of course, FTS do have their limitations, such as sometimes showing a false positive or false negative, only showing binary results, and not being able to test plant products (e.g., marijuana).[10]

The literature focused on the effectiveness of FTS distribution through community-based organizations shows promising results. A 2018 study from North Carolina found that participants who reported a positive FTS result, when compared with those who reported a negative result, were significantly more likely to report a change in drug use behavior, including using less than usual and insufflating instead of injecting.[11] Similarly, a 2018 project from Rhode Island revealed that receiving a positive result was significantly associated with reporting positive changes in overdose risk behavior.[12] Lastly, a recent evaluation of a Wisconsin-based FTS intervention revealed that a positive result was associated with significantly more safe use practices, although this significance was lost when adjusting for age and polysubstance use.[13] AJPH

ABOUT THE AUTHORS

C. Greer McCollum, Greg Ventrelli, Kelly W. Gagnon, and Ellen Eaton are with the Heersink School of Medicine, University of Alabama at Birmingham. Ashley Loftis, Abimbola Famurewa, and Carie Wimberly are with the Addiction Prevention Coalition, Birmingham, AL.

CORRESPONDENCE

Correspondence should be sent to C. Greer McCollum, 41 Levan St, Kingston, NY 12401 (e-mail: gmccollum@uabmc.edu). Reprints can be ordered at https://www.ajph.org by clicking the "Reprints" link.

PUBLICATION INFORMATION

Full Citation: McCollum CG, Ventrelli G, Gagnon KW, et al. Rapid response to the legalization of fentanyl test strips in Alabama: an academic–community partnership. *Am J Public Health*. 2024;114(8):785–788.

Acceptance Date: March 28, 2024.

DOI: https://doi.org/10.2105/AJPH.2024.307681

CONTRIBUTORS

C. G. McCollum visualized the data. C. G. McCollum, G. Ventrelli, K. W. Gagnon, A. Loftis, and E. Eaton wrote the article. C. G. McCollum and A. Famurewa analyzed the data. C. G. McCollum and E. Eaton created the methodology. A. Loftis and A. Famurewa collected the data. C. Wimberly and E. Eaton conceptualized the study and acquired funding. All authors edited the article.

ACKNOWLEDGMENTS

This project was funded by the Substance Abuse and Mental Health Services Administration in 2020 (grant 5H79SP082270-04).

CONFLICTS OF INTEREST

The authors have no conflicts of interest to report.

HUMAN PARTICIPANT PROTECTION

The University of Alabama at Birmingham's institution review board approved this project on December 17, 2020 (IRB-300006219).

REFERENCES

1. Substance Abuse and Mental Health Services Administration. Substance Abuse and HIV Prevention Navigator Program for Racial/Ethnic Minorities. 2021. Available at: https://www.samhsa.gov/grants/grant-announcements/sp-20-001. Accessed May 22, 2024.
2. Centers for Disease Control and Prevention. Evidence-based strategies for preventing opioid overdose: what's working in the United States. 2022. Available at: https://www.oaa.virginia.gov/media/governorvirginiagov/oaa/applications/individual-cityx2fcounties/Stafford-Evidence-Based-Support.pdf. Accessed May 22, 2024.
3. Carson M. Alabama lawmakers pass bill to legalize fentanyl test strips to help prevent overdoses. 2022. Available at: https://www.al.com/news/2022/03/alabama-lawmakers-pass-bill-to-legalize-fentanyl-test-strips-to-help-prevent-overdoses.html. Accessed May 22, 2024.
4. LegiScan. Alabama Senate Bill 168. 2022. Available at: https://legiscan.com/AL/bill/SB168/2022. Accessed May 22, 2024.
5. DanceSafe. Who we are. 2023. Available at: https://dancesafe.org/about-us. Accessed May 22, 2024.
6. Centers for Disease Control and Prevention. Drug overdose mortality by state. 2022. Available at: https://www.cdc.gov/nchs/pressroom/sosmap/drug_poisoning_mortality/drug_poisoning.htm. Accessed May 22, 2024.
7. Ahmad FB, Cisewski JA, Rossen LM, Sutton P. Provisional drug overdose death counts. 2024. Available at: https://www.cdc.gov/nchs/nvss/vsrr/drug-overdose-data.htm. Accessed May 22, 2024.
8. Jefferson County Coroner/Medical Examiner's Office. Annual report: 2022. 2023. Available at: https://www.jccal.org/Sites/Jefferson_County/Documents/Coroner_Medical%20Examiner%20Office/2022%20annual%20report.pdf. Accessed May 22, 2024.
9. Substance Abuse and Mental Health Services Association. MAI substance abuse/HIV prevention initiative prevention navigator grants quick reference guide. 2023. Available at: https://spars.samhsa.gov/content/mai-substance-abusehiv-prevention-initiative-prevention-navigator-grants-quick-reference. Accessed May 22, 2024.
10. Green TC, Park JN, Gilbert M, et al. An assessment of the limits of detection, sensitivity and specificity of three devices for public health–based drug checking of fentanyl in street-acquired samples. *Int J Drug Policy*. 2020;77:102661. https://doi.org/10.1016/j.drugpo.2020.102661
11. Peiper NC, Clarke SD, Vincent LB, Ciccarone D, Kral AH, Zibbell JE. Fentanyl test strips as an opioid overdose prevention strategy: findings from a syringe services program in the Southeastern United States. *Int J Drug Policy*. 2019;63:122–128. https://doi.org/10.1016/j.drugpo.2018.08.007
12. Krieger MS, Goedel WC, Buxton JA, et al. Use of rapid fentanyl test strips among young adults who use drugs. *Int J Drug Policy*. 2018;61:52–58. https://doi.org/10.1016/j.drugpo.2018.09.009
13. Tilhou AS, Zaborek J, Baltes A, Salisbury-Afshar E, Malicki J, Brown R. Differences in drug use behaviors that impact overdose risk among individuals who do and do not use fentanyl test strips for drug checking. *Harm Reduct J*. 2023;20(1):41. https://doi.org/10.1186/s12954-023-00767-0

Engaging School Champions in the Implementation of a Research Study in Historically Marginalized School Communities

Tara Kenworthy LaMarca, PhD, Mileini Campez-Pardo, PhD, Katheryn C. Sauvigné, BS, Gabriela Guevara, MPH, Rose May Fleurime, RN, and Elizabeth R. Pulgaron, PhD

See also Kapadia, p. 769.

Community engagement in research improves uptake of health interventions and health outcomes among marginalized populations. Researchers from school-based health centers serving marginalized communities in Miami, Florida fostered community engagement in COVID-19 research and health education through collaboration with school staff and student "champions" from June 2021 to June 2023. Evaluations completed by champions assessed acceptability, feasibility, and recommendations for improvements. Overall satisfaction was high among champions. We elaborate on lessons learned and future directions for this type of research collaboration. (*Am J Public Health*. 2024;114(8):789–793. https://doi.org/10.2105/AJPH.2024.307711)

AJPH August 2024, Vol. 114, No. 8

The National Institutes for Health–funded Rapid Acceleration of Diagnostics–Underserved Populations (RADx-UP) Return to School initiative centered on increasing students' access to and uptake of COVID-19 testing. The project described here was one of 16 awardees for this initiative. The research team is based at an academic medical center that operates nine school-based health centers (SBHCs) in Title 1 public schools (three high schools, two middle schools, and four elementary schools). These SBHCs primarily serve racially/ethnically minoritized youths and families from communities that experience high levels of immigration, poverty, trauma, and under- or uninsurance. Services span preventative and diagnostic care, chronic disease management, and mental health treatment.

SBHC services were expanded in 2020 to include COVID-19 testing and vaccination. However, during the COVID-19 pandemic, there was a reduction in clinic utilization due to increased absences and remote learning. Therefore, the research team designed and implemented a prospective, multipart research study to elucidate and address the needs related to COVID-19 testing and vaccination within the nine SBHC schools. Considering the well-documented hesitancy of our SBHCs' communities to engage in research with medical institutions,[1–3] novel outreach initiatives were necessary to engage community members in (1) completion of surveys and focus groups centered on examining the perspectives of students, staff, and parents on COVID-19 vaccines and testing[4] and (2) a health intervention to increase COVID-19 knowledge among parents.

INTERVENTION AND IMPLEMENTATION

Initially, the research team created an advisory board of stakeholders in the school community (consisting of a Department of Health employee, a county health funding agency representative, and school district leaders). However, given the tension with the medical community during the early period of the COVID-19 pandemic, we recognized the need to increase engagement with parents, students, and school staff to ensure successful implementation of the study. We also saw an opportunity to empower members of the school community to be active agents in research, rather than simply passive participants. The avenue for engagement that we chose was identification and support of "champions": individuals who "throw [their] weight behind an innovation."[5(p414)] Champions are key factors in implementation frameworks that detail elements needed for quality implementation of innovations.[6,7] In low-income school settings, the presence of health champions is associated with increased uptake of health interventions.[8,9] The study described herein was intended to assess the feasibility and acceptability of involving school staff and student champions in the promotion and implementation of our research endeavors.

School staff were recruited through flyers distributed by school administration. Staff champions facilitated and coordinated research events and data collection, provided feedback on the health education initiative, and liaised with the school community. Tasks were identified by the research team and requested of the champions monthly. Communication was completed informally via in-person meetings, phone, and e-mail.

Student champions were recruited via flyers posted at their schools, school announcements, and referral by school or SBHC staff. Initially piloted with meetings as needed with a small group of students advising on recruitment, outreach, and advertising, the student champions program was formalized in year 2 of the grant, with supplemental funding. In year 2, champions participated in a monthly to bimonthly health education program led by the research team to prepare students to serve as health advocates for the ongoing research study. Meeting topics included public health, health literacy, problem-solving skills, interviewing skills, and careers in health care. Student champions assisted with study recruitment, community outreach, advertisement campaigns, translation of health promotion materials, and administrative support.

The researcher–champion relationship was designed to be reciprocal, with specific benefits to champions in return for the time, resources, and native knowledge they dedicated to the study. Champions were paid monthly: $55 for students and $120 for staff. The research team participated in school events promoted by the champions. Student champions were offered the additional benefit of an end-of-year field trip to the University of Miami medical campus.

At the end of the project period, champions completed demographic surveys, including race, ethnicity, and languages spoken. Additionally, they anonymously evaluated their experiences via open-ended and multiple-choice questions designed by the research staff about the acceptability and feasibility of the champion initiative. All acceptability and feasibility data described here were self-reported by the champions.

PLACE, TIME, AND PERSONS

Staff champions were recruited across nine SBHC schools in Miami-Dade County, Florida. The student champions were recruited in the three high schools. The RADx-UP project period was from June 2021 through June 2023. Champions committed to a minimum of one school year of service.

Staff champions consisted of one to two school staff members (e.g., teachers, administrators, counselors) per school (n = 18), 14 of whom completed the demographic survey. Fifty-one students attended at least one student champion meeting, and 29 of those students completed the demographic survey. Most staff and student champions were female and from racially/ethnically minoritized groups (Table 1).

PURPOSE

We evaluated the acceptability and feasibility of involving school champions (students and staff) as liaisons in the advertisement, recruitment, and implementation of a research study and health intervention about COVID-19 testing and vaccination in their school communities, via champion self-report.

EVALUATION AND ADVERSE EFFECTS

Eleven staff champions completed the program evaluation. Most reported they would recommend being a school champion to colleagues (82%). About half (45.5%) felt they were effective at engaging the school community in the RADx-UP project.

Twenty-nine student champions completed the evaluation. All respondents indicated that they enjoyed the program extremely (57.1%) or very much (42.9%). Most found the program extremely informative (75.0%), with fewer indicating it was very (18.0%) or moderately (7.0%) informative. Finally, most found the information they learned during the program extremely useful (67.9%), with fewer indicating it was very (17.9%), moderately (10.7%), or slightly (3.6%) useful.

See Table 2 for additional insights on acceptability and feasibility from champions.

SUSTAINABILITY

The long-standing infrastructure of the SBHCs, the active involvement and satisfaction of the champions, and the bidirectional relationship between the

TABLE 1— Demographics of Student and Staff Champions: Miami-Dade County, FL, June 2021–June 2023

Characteristics	Students, Median ±SD or No. (%)	Staff, Median ±SD or No. (%)
Age, y	15.9 ±1.2	41.5 ±7.6
Gender		
Female	25 (86.2)	10 (71.4)
Male	4 (13.8)	4 (28.6)
Race/ethnicity		
White	5 (17.2)	5 (35.7)
Black	22 (75.9)	8 (57.1)
Multiracial	1 (3.5)	1 (7.1)
Hispanic	10 (34.5)	6 (42.9)
Familial country of origin		
Chile	0 (0.0)	1 (7.1)
Colombia	1 (3.5)	0 (0.0)
Cuba	0 (0.0)	2 (14.3)
Dominican Republic	1 (3.5)	1 (7.1)
Haiti	19 (65.5)	0 (0.0)
Honduras	2 (6.9)	0 (0.0)
Nicaragua	1 (3.4)	0 (0.0)
Panama	0 (0.0)	1 (7.1)
Bilingual		
Total[a]	23 (79.3)	5 (35.7)
Haitian Creole	15 (51.7)	1 (7.1)
Spanish	8 (27.6)	4 (28.6)
Staff role		
Administrator	. . .	3 (21.4)
Secretary/assistant	. . .	4 (28.6)
Counselor/discipline coordinator	. . .	3 (21.4)
Teacher	. . .	4 (28.6)

Note. The number of student and staff champions was 29 and 14, respectively.
[a]Bilingual included English plus one other language (Haitian Creole or Spanish).

school champions and the research team facilitated sustainability for the champion intervention. However, additional funding strategies outside of reliance on grants would be needed to ensure continued staff support for the educational programming for champions. Further, competing demands on student champions' time affected their participation in the program, suggesting that additional solutions are necessary to ensure active participation. Solutions may include offering transportation or embedding this program in the school curriculum.

PUBLIC HEALTH SIGNIFICANCE

School champions facilitated the research–school partnership among the SBHC team, school personnel, parents, and students in minoritized communities. The champion–researcher partnership empowered members of the school community to influence the response to COVID-19 in their specific school setting. In addition to the potential direct effects of the broader RADx-UP study on public health, the effects of engaging champions—such as the overall positive experience of the champions, the experience of partaking in research, and feeling heard by research staff—may have lasting public health implications yet to be determined (e.g., promoting interest in health care careers). We hope that this Notes From the Field offers a potential model for SBHCs or academic health centers that work with marginalized

TABLE 2— Summary of Student and Staff Responses on the Acceptability and Feasibility of the Champions Initiative: Miami-Dade County, FL, June 2021–June 2023

Themes and Responses	Student Champions, No. (%)	Staff Champions, No. (%)
Barriers to student participation		
Lack of time/competing activities	15 (53.6)	. . .
Lack of transportation	5 (17.9)	. . .
Miscommunication on meeting dates	4 (14.3)	. . .
Personal illness or family issues	3 (10.7)	. . .
Favorite parts of the program/things that went well		
Field trip to the university medical campus	12 (42.9)	. . .
Learning about health care professions from health care professionals	10 (35.7)	3 (27.3)
Assisting with health interventions/research	4 (14.3)	11 (100.0)
Feeling heard	4 (14.3)	7 (63.6)
Payment	2 (7.1)	. . .
Recommended changes to the program		
More field trips	6 (21.4)	1 (9.1)
More interactive activities or more opportunities to contribute	6 (21.4)	4 (36.4)
No specific recommendations	6 (21.4)	. . .
More trainings/discussions on health topics	3 (10.7)	1 (9.1)
Increased communication between researchers and champions through various means including e-mail and other platforms (e.g., group chats)	1 (3.4)	1 (9.1)
Increased advertisement of the research and health endeavors carried out by the team to the school at large	1 (3.4)	6 (54.5)
Change meeting times	2 (7.1)	. . .
Increase frequency of meetings	2 (7.1)	. . .
Higher payment amount or additional tangible incentives (e.g., food or gas)	1 (3.6)	1 (9.1)

Note. The number of student and staff champions was 29 and 11, respectively.

communities to engage and empower community members as partners in research and intervention. AJPH

ABOUT THE AUTHORS

Tara Kenworthy LaMarca, Mileini Campez-Pardo, Katheryn C. Sauvigné, Gabriela Guevara, and Elizabeth R. Pulgaron are with the University of Miami Miller School of Medicine, Miami, FL. Rose May Fleurime is with North Miami Senior High School, North Miami, FL.

CORRESPONDENCE

Correspondence should be sent to Tara Kenworthy LaMarca, PhD, Mailman Center for Child Development, University of Miami Miller School of Medicine, 1601 NW 12th Ave, Miami, FL 33136 (e-mail: tlk38@miami.edu). Reprints can be ordered at https://www.ajph.org by clicking the "Reprints" link.

PUBLICATION INFORMATION

Full Citation: Kenworthy LaMarca T, Campez-Pardo M, Sauvigné KC, Guevara G, Fleurime RM, Pulgaron ER. Engaging school champions in the implementation of a research study in historically marginalized school communities. *Am J Public Health*. 2024;114(8): 789–793.

Acceptance Date: April 20, 2024.

DOI: https://doi.org/10.2105/AJPH.2024.307711

ORCID iD:
Tara Kenworthy LaMarca https://orcid.org/0000-0003-1121-9078

CONTRIBUTORS

T. Kenworthy LaMarca contributed to conceptualization of the study and data collection, wrote the first draft of the article, and critically revised the article. M. Campez-Pardo contributed to conceptualization of the study and data collection, conducted statistical analysis, and contributed to the writing, interpretation, and revision of the article. K. Sauvigné conducted statistical analysis and contributed to the writing, interpretation, and revision of the article. G. Guevara contributed to the writing, interpretation, and revision of the article. R. M. Fleurime participated in the project as a community partner and contributed to interpretation and revision. E. R. Pulgaron supervised the study, contributed to the conceptualization of the study, and contributed to the writing, interpretation, and revision of the article.

ACKNOWLEDGMENTS

Research reported in this Rapid Acceleration of Diagnostics–Underserved Populations (RADx-UP) publication was supported by the National Institutes of Health (award no. OT2HD108111).

We thank all student and staff champions for taking part in this initiative.

Note. The views and opinions herein are those of the individual authors and do not necessarily represent those of the NIH.

CONFLICTS OF INTEREST

The authors have no conflicts of interest to disclose.

HUMAN PARTICIPANT PROTECTION

This study was exempt from institutional review board oversight at the University of Miami because it is a program evaluation.

REFERENCES

1. Martinez CR Jr, McClure HH, Eddy JM, Ruth B, Hyers MJ. Recruitment and retention of Latino immigrant families in prevention research. *Prev Sci.* 2012;13(1):15–26. https://doi.org/10.1007/s11121-011-0239-0
2. Metellus G, Hilaire S, Hermantin L, Lacroix S. *Risk and Protective Factors in Little Haiti and in the Haitian/Haitian American Community in Miami-Dade County.* Miami, FL: Sant La; 2004.
3. Shedlin MG, Decena CU, Mangadu T, Martinez A. Research participant recruitment in Hispanic communities: lessons learned. *J Immigr Minor Health.* 2011;13(2):352–360.
4. Kenworthy T, Harmon SL, Delouche A, et al. Community voices on factors influencing COVID-19 concerns and health decisions among racial and ethnic minorities in the school setting. *Front Public Health.* 2022;10:1002209. https://doi.org/10.3389/fpubh.2022.1002209
5. Rogers EM. *Diffusion of Innovations.* 5th ed. New York, NY: Free Press; 2003.
6. Damschroder LJ, Aron DC, Keith RE, Kirsh SR, Alexander JA, Lowery JC. Fostering implementation of health services research findings into practice: a consolidated framework for advancing implementation science. *Implement Sci.* 2009;4(1):50. https://doi.org/10.1186/1748-5908-4-50
7. Scaccia JP, Cook BS, Lamont A, et al. A practical implementation science heuristic for organizational readiness: R = MC^2. *J Community Psychol.* 2015;43(4):484–501. https://doi.org/10.1002/jcop.21698
8. Lucarelli JF, Alaimo K, Mang E, et al. Facilitators to promoting health in schools: is school health climate the key? *J Sch Health.* 2014;84(2):133–140. https://doi.org/10.1111/josh.12123
9. Naylor PJ, Macdonald HM, Zebedee JA, Reed KE, McKay HA. Lessons learned from Action Schools! BC–an "active school" model to promote physical activity in elementary schools. *J Sci Med Sport.* 2006;9(5):413–423. https://doi.org/10.1016/j.jsams.2006.06.013

Business, Ventilation, and Health—Can We Have Them All?

Melanie A. Kiechle, PhD

ABOUT THE AUTHOR

Melanie A. Kiechle is with the Department of History, Virginia Polytechnic Institute and State University, Blacksburg.

See also Indoor Air Quality & Public Health, pp. 796–804.

In his opening comments at the 2022 White House Summit on Indoor Air Quality, Ashish Jha, MD, MPH, the White House's COVID-19 response coordinator, reflected on the history of public health advances. Jha explained that when waterborne pathogens were understood, "we learned that you could of course boil your water and make it safer, but the policy solution was not everybody should boil their water all the time." Instead, a series of policy changes and systematic engineering efforts improved the healthfulness and safety of drinking water, curbing the spread of the gastrointestinal ailments that once dominated mortality charts. Jha pivoted from this public health achievement to say, "Indoor air is the next frontier when it comes to thinking about public health."[1]

Indoor air is not a new topic for public health. Jha's comments echoed New York City physician and public health advocate John Hoskins Griscom Jr., who opened his 1852 public lecture on ventilation by talking about water safety. According to the *New York Times*:

> Dr. Griscom commenced his lecture by observing that the importance of pure air was not so much studied as it ought to be, or it would be the care of persons generally to obtain as much purity in the atmosphere of their dwellings as possible. The City of New-York had spent fifteen million dollars in endeavoring to obtain pure water, but this was not more necessary to health and life than was pure air.[2(p1)]

Griscom frequently compared the city's immense expenditures to secure safe drinking water (more than $600 million in today's currency) with its failure to invest in ventilation. If New York City's citizens wanted to protect health, Griscom argued, they should invest in both water and air quality. For Griscom, as for many other 19th-century sanitarians, improving the whole environment was the best method for preventing disease. Yet governments and business leaders invested in environmental changes that would directly benefit businesses. Many businesses benefited from increased water supplies, but sewer systems that carried away excess water and human waste lagged behind because their "revenue-generating potential was limited."[3(p62)] Sewer systems curbed the spread of cholera and gastrointestinal illnesses but were adopted slowly because sewers were not directly profitable.

Is the profit motive why, in the face of respiratory diseases that are transmitted through the air we breathe, so many ventilation proponents emphasize outcomes other than disease prevention? As LaFay and Sampson document in "Ventilation and Public Health: A Fraught History" (p. 798 in this issue of *AJPH*), many of the recent justifications for improving ventilation have emphasized increased worker productivity and student performance. Both were talking points at the White House Summit.

LaFay and Sampson's history of ventilation efforts demonstrates how leaving a public health necessity to private development has created health inequities that follow social inequality. Ship ventilation did not protect enslaved men and women from the deadly effects of overcrowding, poor nutrition, and abuse. Similarly, windows and air shafts could not combat the vermin and fires that killed tenement dwellers. Nor could HVAC (heating, ventilation, and air-conditioning) systems combat the neurologic effects of chemicals emitted from new building materials in postwar airtight high-rise offices. Ventilation and indoor air quality, when removed from the comprehensive environmental improvements that 19th-century sanitarians sought, have not prevented illness and death.

These failures of ventilation do not mean that we should abandon the effort. Instead, LaFay and Sampson argue, ventilation should be integrated into social and health policies. Better ventilation will curb the spread of respiratory diseases. In addition, ventilation should be pursued through the same avenues that gave modern society safe drinking water.

In his opening comments at the White House Summit, Jha demonstrates his understanding of the history of public health advances, but he ignores that laws and regulations

AJPH August 2024, Vol. 114, No. 8

created our healthy water supply. The White House Summit on Indoor Air Quality did not launch equivalent policy changes and systematic engineering efforts to improve the safety of the air that those who live in the United States inhale in homes and public buildings. Instead, the summit promoted the Environmental Protection Agency's Clean Air in Buildings Challenge, a voluntary "pledge opportunity" that invites businesses and building owners to commit publicly to improving indoor air quality.[4] The challenge is the latest in a long history of public health initiatives that are business friendly.

When Griscom advocated ventilation in 19th-century New York City, he also learned to be business friendly. This meant focusing his ire on sublandlords rather than the landowners who were responsible for the exploitative real estate system in which buildings were overcrowded and undermaintained.[5]

New York City tried to improve ventilation through a series of Tenement House Acts passed between 1867 and 1901 that stipulated room size, number of windows, and the proportion of the lot that buildings could occupy. Rather than adhere to these regulations, landowners maximized rentable living space by adopting architect James Ware's "dumbbell tenement." Even when public health regulations have tried to curb businesses in favor of health, businesspeople have found ways to make money, often at the expense of public health.

Unlike the history of ventilation, the history of the water supply in the United States is thick with laws, ordinances, and regulations. Early public health departments tested water and published reports that led to standards and regulations. Massachusetts passed laws preventing pollution and permitting experiments on water purification in the 1880s.[6] In the early 20th century, as it became evident that filtration could remove bacteria, cities adopted filtration systems.

Since the creation of the Environmental Protection Agency in 1974, the United States has had national standards that protect public drinking water and its sources.[7] Economists have found that the Clean Water Act and the Safe Drinking Water Act have been effective in reducing water pollution.[8] None of these standards has been promoted as challenges. Instead, the history of water supplies in the United States is one of engineering efforts, scientific analyses, and legal regulations with which individuals and businesses have had to comply.

Should we want to learn from the past, we need to know not only what changes have improved public health but also how those changes were implemented. Laws and regulations have accomplished more than voluntary appeals to business leaders and building owners. AJPH

CORRESPONDENCE

Correspondence should be sent to Melanie A. Kiechle, 431 Major Williams Hall (0117), 220 Stanger St, Blacksburg, VA 24061 (e-mail: mkiechle@vt.edu). Reprints can be ordered at https://www.ajph.org by clicking the "Reprints" link.

PUBLICATION INFORMATION

Full Citation: Kiechle MA. Business, ventilation, and health—can we have them all? *Am J Public Health*. 2024;114(8):794–795.

Acceptance Date: May 9, 2024.

DOI: https://doi.org/10.2105/AJPH.2024.307727

ORCID iD:
Melanie A. Kiechle https://orcid.org/0000-0001-9516-7978

ACKNOWLEDGMENTS

The author thanks Dennis Patrick Halpin and Kara Murphy Schlichting for their suggestions and feedback, as well as Elaine LaFay and Paul E. Sampson for writing about the history of ventilation failures.

CONFLICTS OF INTEREST

The author has no conflicts of interest to declare.

REFERENCES

1. Jha A. White House Summit on Indoor Air Quality. October 11, 2022. Available at: https://www.youtube.com/watch?v=1BeEfDLDJSA. Accessed May 31, 2024.
2. Lectures for the people: the importance of proper ventilation. *New York Times*. January 21, 1852, 1.
3. Melosi MV. *The Sanitary City: Environmental Services in Urban America From Colonial Times to the Present*. Abridged ed. Pittsburgh, PA: University of Pittsburgh Press; 2008.
4. White House. Clean air in buildings: pledge opportunity. Available at: https://www.whitehouse.gov/cleanindoorair. Accessed April 25, 2024.
5. Blackmar E. Accountability for public health: regulating the housing market of nineteenth-century New York City. In: Rosner D, ed. *Hives of Sickness: Public Health and Epidemics in New York City*. New Brunswick, NJ: Rutgers University Press; 1995:42–64.
6. Rosenkrantz BG. *Public Health and the State: Changing View in Massachusetts, 1842–1936*. Cambridge, MA: Harvard University Press; 1972.
7. Centers for Disease Control and Prevention. History of drinking water regulations. Available at: https://archive.cdc.gov/#/details?q=https://www.cdc.gov/healthywater/surveillance/drinking-water-reg-history.html&start=0&rows=10&url=https://www.cdc.gov/healthywater/surveillance/drinking-water-reg-history.html. Accessed May 3, 2024.
8. Keiser DA, Shapiro JS. US water pollution regulation over the past half century: burning waters to Crystal Springs? *J Econ Perspect*. 2019;33(4):51–75. https://doi.org/10.1257/jep.33.4.51

The "Best of All Breathing"?

Christopher Hamlin, PhD

ABOUT THE AUTHOR

Christopher Hamlin is professor emeritus with the Department of History and the Program in the History and Philosophy of Science, University of Notre Dame, Notre Dame, IN.

See also Indoor Air Quality & Public Health, pp. 794–804.

Novelist William Faulkner's magnificent phrase applies to far fewer people than it should.[1] Historians are partly responsible for that. Maybe they can help to fix it.

LaFay and Sampson (p. 798) in this issue of *AJPH* rightly call air's status in public health history "fraught." Concern with occasional adventitious constituents has been hard to translate into sensibilities about exposure or prophylaxis. For arthropod vectors or for water, it is easier. A leader in 19th-century medical hygiene in the United Kingdom, John Snow's famous map lets us follow water from a single well to containers, guts, excretions, and new cholera cases. But air? Molecules leap from surfaces, are exuded by beings, go up chimneys. They ignore channels, never find sinks. Some harm health, but dodging them is hard when you cannot see the medium or what it carries. And airs have incidental properties affecting well-being: temperature, moisture, and movement. I know when water wets, but air always aerates.[2] No one gets away with the "I don't inhale" excuse for long. And if we live under a sea of air, surely we should be swimming. A mysterious "air handler" lives in the furnace. Good thing—*I* can't *handle* air.

Although students introduced to Hippocrates's *Airs, Waters, Places* usually fixate on the water, airs have loomed much larger in health anxieties; we need only think of mal-air-ia, which was a geographic descriptor before becoming a disease.

Historians, sometimes using "miasma" to stand in for bad science, have been coconspirators with consolidators of professional public health in the relegation of "air" to "error." Emphasis on acute diseases and visible public undertakings with big payoffs helped public health to establish itself and garner public support but also shaped the field in terms of core and periphery.[3] Had architects, urban planners, or engineers led the professionalization, matters of air would have been more central, yet the shape of public health (and of those professions) would be different.

But it is hard to respond rationally to what you cannot see. Current air-mindedness reflects the shock of COVID-19. Who knew that sharing air with other droplet-dropping or aerosol-emitting exhalers showing no stigmata of danger could kill you? Or that you could kill them? Air hygiene often must operate in the realm of imagination simply because we cannot perceive air quality. Early in the pandemic, before the call to mask, I handled my fear by doubling over a welder's hat and sewing on an elastic band. It was snug (I could barely breathe), and knowing that welders worked in dangerous airs reassured me, if unreasonably. To the micron-minded, my efforts were primitive and pathetic, yet as many of us discovered, the sleek, sharp, N95s did not eliminate anxiety; they might have magnified it. For me, doing my best put my mind at ease.

Air anxiety is not new. Go back two millennia and we find air as the first of Greco-Roman physician Galen's six things nonnatural, factors physicians adjust to manage health. "You need a change of air," they say.[4]

Or pop ahead to the 1740s to John Pringle, expert on army air. He confronted a problem that persists: is outdoor air better than indoor? He worried about soldiers sleeping on damp ground but more about "effluvia" from sick and wounded bodies in hospitals.[5] The great fix of moving air, ventilation, was often unpopular. Laypersons, having "caught a draft," would blanket themselves in closed spaces, but Pringle would have the draft catch the patient. Later one hears of medics breaking windows to expel the fetid air and expose the ill body to a cleansing wind. Nursing manuals would extol the sash window, which must be pulled down from the top and up from the bottom.[6,7] My parents, raised to view fresh air as a panacea, insisted that my bedroom window be open a crack even on January nights with temperatures reaching −30° Fahrenheit. (Later, amid the energy crisis, I would turn to the opposite extreme, a fanatic with tape and caulk, futilely seeking out cracks.)

Air paranoia peaked in the mid-19th–century heyday of English sanitarianism. The great undertaking of the hydraulic city (good water in, wastes washed out) began as a way to fix the air infected with all that might stink. The greatest paranoia was with reflux: what went down the sewers might bubble back as imperceptible "sewer gas" unless trapped by a water seal or sent harmlessly over the roofs by a vent pipe. Want a challenging historical project? Try mastering Victorian trap design debates.[8] Acceptance of the "zymotic" diseases (those presumed to result from decay) as spread by ingestion rather than inhalation was slow, both in public health science and lay sensibility, but was a hallmark of the progress associated with John Snow and German microbiologist Robert Koch.

At the same time, a sanitarian public health often marginalized not only respiratory infections, most conspicuously tuberculosis, but indoor matters: dwellings and workplaces. Often these were public, yet not unambiguously public health, matters. Not only were sewers public in a way that sleeping spaces were not, the latter were more clearly subject to the invidious tradeoffs at the nexus of lifeboat ethics and slave ship economics that Karl Marx recognized: the equating of space with life and money.[9]

Later 19th-century campaigns to regulate occupancy had mixed motivations. Worries about morality and generic concern with contagion are more prominent, but ventilation, sometimes conceived as adequate respiration, is the proxy susceptible to regulation: inspectors unable to measure throughput might insist on windows or on minimum cubic feet per person; yet in enforcing occupancy limits in the name of public health, they neglected to confront the question of which person is the extra who must leave the lifeboat, if only to climb into another.[10,11]

Public health was no match for a labor market requiring people to live near their work. Cold exacerbated crowdedness. A stove must have a draft, but better to keep all heat, even if it means keeping exhaust gases. Surely there were many deaths from CO, though its toxicity was elucidated only in 1856.[12] Workplaces brought similar issues, with the addition of heat, dust, and trade toxins and ventilation often seen as interfering with quality control.

We may be surprised that ventilation acquired any priority. Economies favored filling space with blocks of building. Even so, windows would be for opening as well as light, and ventilation would become standard in urban building design. Urban planners would straighten streets to facilitate the cleansing wind. They would build parks. We find such agendas in late 19th-century public health manuals; nonetheless, around 1900, the "new" case and germ–tracking public health generally left them as someone else's business.[13] That would carry over to the new technology of air conditioning. Heat emergencies requiring cooling stations are becoming common, yet in public health history air conditioning registers mainly as the medium of legionnaires disease.

The United Nations recognizes rights to water and sanitation. But air? Inequalities exist; they register as harm to health. Are they violations of rights? Indoor and outdoor airs are regulated by governments or standard-setting professional bodies. In the wake of COVID-19 the World Health Organization has taken up the issue.[14] Still, concepts of fair breathing will ultimately require changed sensibilities. Had COVID-19 been a fecal–oral disease, concerted action would have been much easier. The golden rule and 18th-century philosopher Immanuel Kant's categorical imperative work for excretions. Perhaps they might work for exhalations, letting us give to one another more gifts of good air. AJPH

CORRESPONDENCE

Correspondence should be sent to Christopher Hamlin, Professor Emeritus, University of Notre Dame, 919 Oak Ridge Dr, South Bend, IN 46617 (e-mail: chamlin@nd.edu). Reprints can be ordered at https://www.ajph.org by clicking the "Reprints" link.

PUBLICATION INFORMATION

Full Citation: Hamlin C. The "best of all breathing"? *Am J Public Health*. 2024;114(8):796–797.

Acceptance Date: May 21, 2024.

DOI: https://doi.org/10.2105/AJPH.2024.307735

CONFLICTS OF INTEREST

The author has no conflicts of interest to disclose.

REFERENCES

1. Faulkner W. The bear. In: *Go Down Moses*. New York, NY: Random House; 1942:191–334.
2. Christopher Hamlin. Wet dirt: a phenomenological-historical foundation for green sanitation as environmental justice. *City and Environment Interactions*. 2023;17:100092. https://doi.org/10.1016/j.cacint.2022.100092
3. Winslow C-EA. *The Conquest of Epidemic Disease*. Princeton, NJ: Princeton University Press; 1943.
4. Jarcho S. Galen's six non-naturals: a bibliographic note and translation. *Bull Hist Med*. 1970;44(4):372–377.
5. Pringle J. *Observations on the Diseases of the Army in Camp and Garrison*. London: Millar, Wilson and Payne; 1752.
6. Register EC. *Practical Fever Nursing*. Philadelphia, PA: W. B. Saunders; 1907.
7. Paul GP. *Nursing in the Acute Infectious Fevers*. Philadelphia, PA: W. B. Saunders; 1906.
8. Moore ECS. *Sanitary Engineering; A Practical Treatise on the Collection, Removal and Final Disposal of Sewage*, . . . New York, NY: Longmans; 1898.
9. Marx K. *Capital: A Critical Analysis of Capitalist Production*. Moore S, Aveling E, trans. New York: International Publishing; 1939:I.149–150.
10. Wohl A. *The Eternal Slum: Housing and Social Policy in Victorian London*. London: Edward Arnold; 1977.
11. Hamlin C. Nuisances and community in mid-Victorian England: the attractions of inspection. *Soc Hist*. 2013;38(3):346–379. https://doi.org/10.1080/03071022.2013.817061
12. Sternbach GL, Varon J. Claude Bernard: on the origin of carbon monoxide poisoning. *Resuscitation*. 2003;58(2):127–130. https://doi.org/10.1016/S0300-9572(03)00213-2
13. Hamlin C. The city as a chemical system? The chemist as urban environmental professional in France and Britain, 1780–1880. *J Urban Hist*. 2007;33(5):702–728. https://doi.org/10.1177/0096144207301416
14. World Health Organization. Roadmap to improve and ensure good indoor ventilation in the context of COVID-19. Available at: https://www.who.int/publications-detail-redirect/9789240021280. Accessed May 13, 2024.

Ventilation and Public Health: A Fraught History

Elaine LaFay, PhD, and Paul Sampson, PhD

See also Indoor Air Quality & Public Health, pp. 794–797.

Since the beginning of the COVID-19 pandemic, a vigorous public health discussion has arisen over indoor air quality and ventilation. In popular press articles, bestselling books, and the US Environmental Protection Agency's recently announced Clean Air in Buildings Challenge, scholars and policy experts have claimed that improved ventilation systems can lead to better productivity and performance. By reevaluating those claims in light of the history of public health in Great Britain and the United States, we found that better ventilation has frequently been proposed as a cost-effective and nonintrusive means of improving health in institutions experiencing structural and environmental public health problems. Furthermore, our examination of efforts to provide ventilation for enslaved people, incarcerated people, and the urban poor revealed a consistent lack of government regulation and a disassociation of air quality concerns from broader environmental, social, and economic realities. By continuing to ignore these broader contexts, current ventilation efforts risk repeating this pattern. (*Am J Public Health.* 2024;114(8):798–804. https://doi.org/10.2105/AJPH.2024.307670)

AJPH August 2024, Vol. 114, No. 8

Ventilation has been in the air recently. Well-founded fears of airborne disease have created an atmosphere of concern about air quality in workplaces, schools, and homes. Since the beginning of the COVID-19 pandemic, a gust of editorials advocating improved ventilation have appeared in the *New York Times*, *Forbes*, and *Time* magazine, as well as in *Scientific American* and the *Harvard Business Review*.[1]

Although the impetus for these efforts has clearly been to address the airborne spread of the novel coronavirus, the focus of this discourse has been to improve ventilation to boost productivity and academic performance. An editorial in *The Economist* titled "Fresh Thinking About Fresh Air" claims that "cognitive scores of people in well-ventilated offices are 61% higher than those of workers in conventional office set-ups."[2] In their award-winning 2020 book *Healthy Buildings: How Indoor Spaces Drive Performance and Productivity*, environmental expert Joseph G. Allen and former real-estate CEO John D. Macomber argued that the condition of indoor air influences productivity: "When we make our buildings healthy, we make the people in those buildings healthier and more productive, and that translates into a healthier bottom line."[3]

The Biden administration has been proactive in responding to these calls. In March 2022, the Environmental Protection Agency launched the Clean Air in Buildings Challenge, which included new guidance for "optimizing fresh air ventilation."[4] In a virtual event titled "Let's Clear the Air on COVID," Alondra Nelson, head of the White House Office of Science and Technology Policy, linked improved ventilation to past environmental initiatives: "For decades Americans have demanded that clean water flow from our taps and pollution limits to be placed on our smokestacks and tailpipes, and our indoor air should be clean and healthy too."[5]

Nelson's reference to past public health initiatives is echoed in an editorial in *The Economist*, which compares the emerging focus on ventilation with the pioneering work of Victorian sanitary reformer Edwin Chadwick, who "showed that poor sanitation was associated with poor health" and "lifted people's expectations that the water coming out of their taps would be clean."[6]

However, many popular examples drawn from the 19th century "sanitary revolution" reveal a simplified view of the history of public health. The successes of the sanitary revolution in improving sewerage and access to clean water entailed enormous public investments in improving the quality of sewerage and drinking water.[7] By focusing public efforts on sanitation and leaving health necessities such as ventilation, nutrition, shelter, and medical care to the private sphere, Victorian public health advocates assured businesses that it was possible to improve public health and empower the free market at the same time.[8] The result was that although water quality drastically improved, air pollution in London continued to be a major public health hazard well into the 20th century.[9]

Contemporary advocates of ventilation risk repeating the same mistake. Although fresh, clean air is rightly viewed as essential for health, most attempts to improve ventilation have been privately led, underfunded, and promoted on the basis of improving economic productivity. As a result, in the words of two public health historians, poor air quality infrastructure has been "built into the urban environment over generations."[10] The repeated failures of ventilation efforts in Great Britain and the United States reveal that wealth and social status often determine access to fresh air.

EARLY HISTORY OF VENTILATION

In the long history of ventilation, air and politics have frequently intermingled. Since the time of the Ancient Roman author Vitruvius, architects considered "natural ventilation," or the positioning of windows and doorways to receive healthy breezes, a priority for healthy buildings. Prevailing medical wisdom also emphasized the body's need for fresh air. Following the ancient Hippocratic "airs, waters, places" tradition, doctors argued that air and climate strongly influenced bodily composition, health, and character.[11] Some physicians even argued that national character was determined by the aerial environment. "The genius of nations depends on that of their air,"[12] wrote British polymath and physician John Arbuthnot in 1733.

Just as fresh air preserved health, foul-smelling and fetid air bred disease. This "miasmatic" model of disease held that heavy respiration and rotting organic matter imbued the air with noxious "effluvias."[13] In 18th-century Great Britain, this problem received public attention as urban populations grew and overseas trade expanded. In ships, factories, and prisons, more and more people were crowded into dank and airless spaces. The predictable results were frequent outbreaks of typhus, which became colloquially known as "ship-fever," "jail fever," or "hospital fever."[14]

Physicians and natural philosophers (the early form of scientists) responded with a spate of proposals to freshen the air in these institutions. The foremost of these were clergyman and inventor Stephen Hales, who, after hearing of a typhus epidemic aboard naval ships, developed a "ventilator trunk" as a means of preventing further outbreaks (Figure 1). These hand-cranked wooden bellows drew in air and blew out foul vapors, thus serving as, in Hales's words, "the Lungs of a Ship." Hales claimed that institutions' use of his ventilator trunk would both save lives and increase labor productivity. By reducing the number of sick and dying sailors, ventilators would prove "a great advantage to navigation" and "traffick [trade] will thereby be much inlarged."[15]

Following Hales's commercial logic, the first uses of his machines were on slave ships. Early adopters, such as slave ship captain Henry Ellis, wrote glowing reviews: the machines were "good exercise for our slaves,"[16] who were "very sensible of the benefits of constant ventilation."[17] However, despite these precautions, mortality among enslaved Africans remained stubbornly high. Surgeons' logs attributed most onboard deaths to fever and gastrointestinal diseases, but other causes included insurrection, suicide, and accidents as enslaved people struggled against their captors.[18]

The pressing dangers to the health of enslaved people were clearly not related to ventilation but to the fundamental inequities created by the slave system. Despite the obvious failure of ventilating devices to prevent inhumanity and disease, proslavery voices insisted that the key to success lay in reforming the air rather than abolishing the institution. In response, antislavery advocates insisted that despite "every comfort, which room, air, variety of nourishment, and careful cleanliness can yield," the hold of a slave ship would always be a "scene of wretchedness."[19]

A similar dynamic played out in efforts to reform and ventilate British prisons. As urban populations grew, more and more incarcerated persons were crammed into filthy, makeshift jails. Debtors were imprisoned alongside violent felons, and all were subjected to the same risk of typhus and smallpox. As public sympathy grew for the many debtors dying in jail, the British Parliament passed the 1774 Act for Preserving the Health of Prisoners. This act stated that disease was caused by the "want of cleanliness and fresh air" and mandated that prisons be "constantly supplied with fresh air, by means of hand ventilators or otherwise."[20] However, these adjustments proved deeply unpopular with incarcerated persons. Annoyed by the constant cold air, incarcerated persons frequently blocked the vents with rags and straw.[21] An inspection of Cold Bath Fields prison in London found that newly

AJPH August 2024, Vol. 114, No. 8

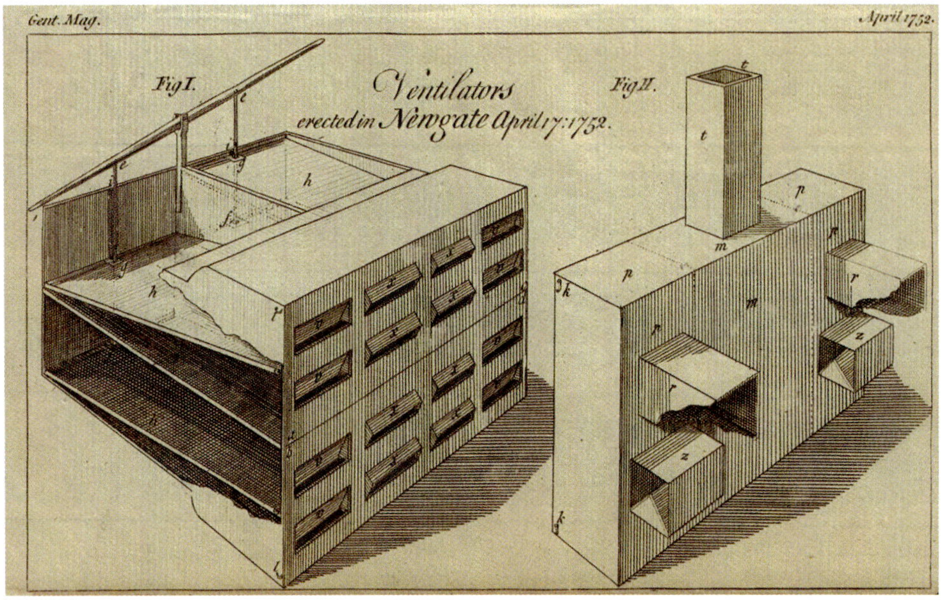

FIGURE 1— Stephen Hales's Ventilator Trunk

Note. This ventilator was designed to expel foul air and take in fresh air through the valves on the front of the device (left). These valves were connected to outside air and the prison wards via the ducts shown on the right.
Source. *Gentleman's Magazine*, 22 (April 1752): 179–182.

installed ventilation shutters had been destroyed in more than 70 of the cells.[22]

By the end of the 18th century, once-optimistic reformers were frustrated that efforts to improve air quality were being undermined by resistance against the oppressive and violent institutions they were trying to ventilate. The next generation of prison reformers shifted tactics to create the modern "penitentiary," an institution designed to ensure discipline through work and moral instruction.[23] To prevent disease, opined naval reformer Gilbert Blane, ventilation and cleanliness would have to be impressed on the public as "moral and religious duties."[24]

VENTILATION AND PUBLIC HEALTH

By the 19th century, ventilation became one of many strategies for improving health in urban environments. As urban reformers fought foul external environments and associated miasma with sanitary interventions such as sewerage construction, they simultaneously turned their attention to remedying foul internal environments through ventilation and other hygienic building improvements. Although it received less attention and funding than large-scale campaigns to drain marshy ground (often necessary for agricultural land development), install sewerage, and remove "filth," ventilation's importance in sanitary frameworks went nearly unquestioned. In 1835, one popular domestic medical guide proclaimed, "No consideration of economy should prevent the most constant attention being paid to proper ventilation, so essential is the latter to health and comfort."[25]

The conviction that miasma caused disease continued to persuade leading epidemiologists, such as William Farr, who interpreted statistical studies of disease to support the idea that air influenced mortality.[26] Alongside miasma, physicians also began to realize the dangers of "carbonic acid gas," or carbon dioxide, which polluted the air with every breath. Some public health experts claimed they could smell this "vitiated air" when CO_2 was at high concentrations.[27] These concerns strongly influenced hospital design. Florence Nightingale, for example, recommended locating hospitals in areas near fresh, open air. "The very first canon of nursing," she emphasized, was "TO KEEP THE AIR [THE PATIENT] BREATHES AS PURE AS THE EXTERNAL AIR."[28]

Whether the cause of disease was miasma or "vitiated air," nearly everyone agreed that ventilation was a powerful tool for addressing airborne disease.[29] Edwin Chadwick declared that "the annual loss of life from filth and bad ventilation are greater than the loss from death or wounds in any wars in which the country has been engaged in modern times."[30] Chadwick's efforts influenced legislation by Great Britain's Parliament, including the Public Health Act (1848) and the establishment of boards of health, each of which included provisions on the ventilation of workplaces, institutions, and homes, especially the homes of the poor.

But bourgeoisie attention to ventilation was animated as much by self-interest as genuine concern. Clean air even became a private commodity as countless advertisements for "ventilating stoves" and "window ventilators" urged homeowners to invest in devices to shield them from the smoky, polluted air outside.[31] An 1853 report in New York City positioned ventilation as one of several ways of preventing the "poisonous miasma" of the poor from reaching "the rich," making ventilation "one of the most interesting and useful efforts of benevolence."[32] Alongside its immediate physical consequences for health, ventilation appealed to physicians and other reformers as part of a moralizing health crusade focused on the working classes.

Language surrounding ventilation was thick with disgust, and bourgeoisie reformers habitually correlated poor ventilation and overcrowding with filth and immorality. Reformers believed that the famously underventilated tenements, which the 1853 report called "filthy and wretched to the extreme," further induced "disease, lower[ed] moral character, and [took] away all thrift and care for decency and cleanliness."[33] Ventilation became an avenue for the bourgeoisie to articulate their profound distaste for the working classes, illustrating the deep social roots of health and hygiene (Figure 2).

Legislative attempts to mandate adequate ventilation in slums were often undermined by profiteering landlords. Beginning in the 1860s, the state of New York passed a series of Tenement House Acts, which were intended to improve living conditions by mandating windows, regulating room size, and requiring access to a fire escape. Landlords found many loopholes in these requirements. The most common solution was the construction of what became known as "dumbbell tenements," apartment buildings with a legally required three-foot-wide air shaft in the middle. To save money, landlords argued that these narrow spaces were adequate for all sanitary requirements and neglected to build drains or chimneys. The ventilation shafts quickly filled with waste and bilge water and smoke, ironically becoming a source of foul air rather than an outlet.[34] Meanwhile, physicians and public health reformers continued to lay the blame for poor

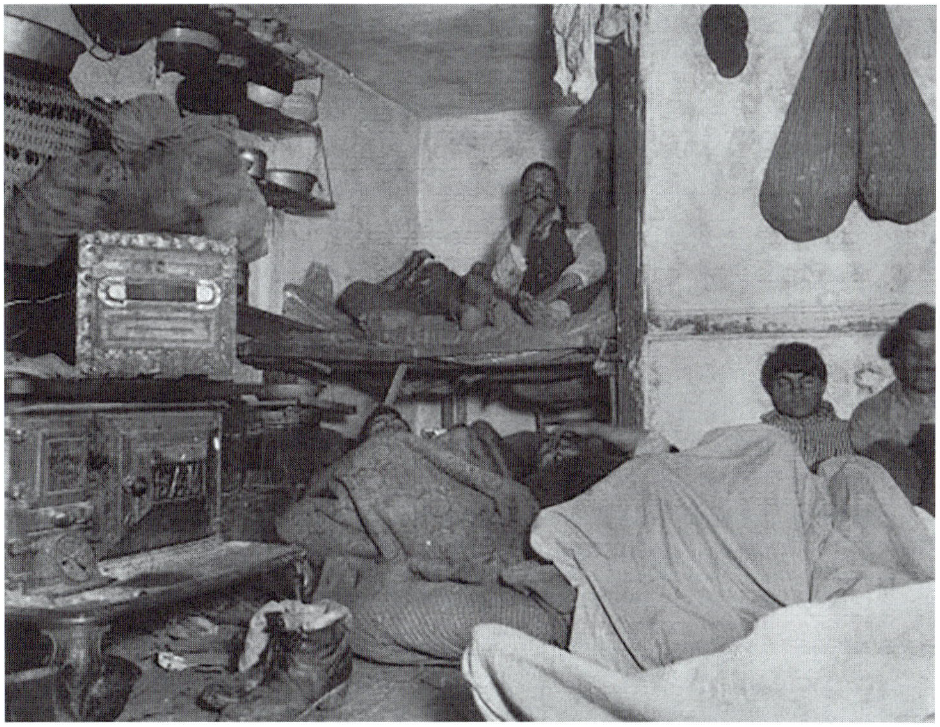

FIGURE 2— "Lodgers in Bayard Street Tenement, Five Cents a Spot," Jacob Riis, 1889

Note. Reformers like Jacob Riis used images like this one of a shelter for immigrants to illustrate the poorly ventilated and dimly lit rooms that characterized tenement housing. Note the absence of windows and ventilation of any kind.
Source. Jacob Riis, *How the Other Half Lives: Studies Among the Tenements of New York* (New York, NY: Charles Scribner's Sons, 1914, 69).

ventilation on individual tenants while eliding the social and political realities underpinning such living conditions.

VENTILATION AND PRODUCTIVITY

Just as Allen and Macomber advocated in *Healthy Buildings*, Victorians also saw ventilation as a means of improving productivity. However, they were divided on how ventilation fit with other social concerns. On one side, socialists and public health experts argued that working conditions could make a person sick. Public health expert Rudolf Virchow, who studied outbreaks of typhus in Silesia, argued that the cause of epidemics was "defects in our social system."[35] In his study of the working class in Manchester, Great Britan, Friedrich Engels quoted a physician who claimed that "the absence of all appropriate regulations for ventilation and cleanliness in the mills very decidedly [is] the chief cause"[36] of worker deaths. These authors believed that public health strategies such as ventilation could only operate alongside higher wages, improved working and living conditions, access to food, and other political interventions.

But Chadwick and his followers maintained that sanitation and politics were separate pursuits. His formulation was simple and apolitical: remove filth, and disease will be eradicated.[37] Thus public health became devoted to sanitation, ventilation, and the removal of filth, ignoring other important aspects of health such as social and working conditions. Chadwick's program animated the pursuit of ventilation in the service of hygiene, with an eye fixed on labor.

There was also a growing tendency to view labor issues as scientific problems. By the late 19th century, scientific studies on fatigue furthered the view of laborers as machines whose needs could be measured, predicted, and calibrated.[38] By the 1910s and 1920s, ventilation was part of an industrial project of reducing fatigue; perhaps, experts argued, workers would labor faster with fresher air.[39] Improving working conditions through ventilation remained a project of increasing labor output.[40]

By the mid-20th century, chemicals from carpets, building materials, adhesives, solvents, and other seemingly hidden risky materials shifted the conversation on health and ventilation from fresh air to chemical exposure. In the 1980s, an epidemic of "sick building syndrome" challenged previous understandings of health in the built environment. Unlike noxious smells or miasma, chemical toxicity was largely imperceptible. The accumulation of toxic hazards left office workers, many of them women, with conditions ranging from headaches, rashes, and fatigue to life-threatening cancers (Figure 3).[41] Air inspectors

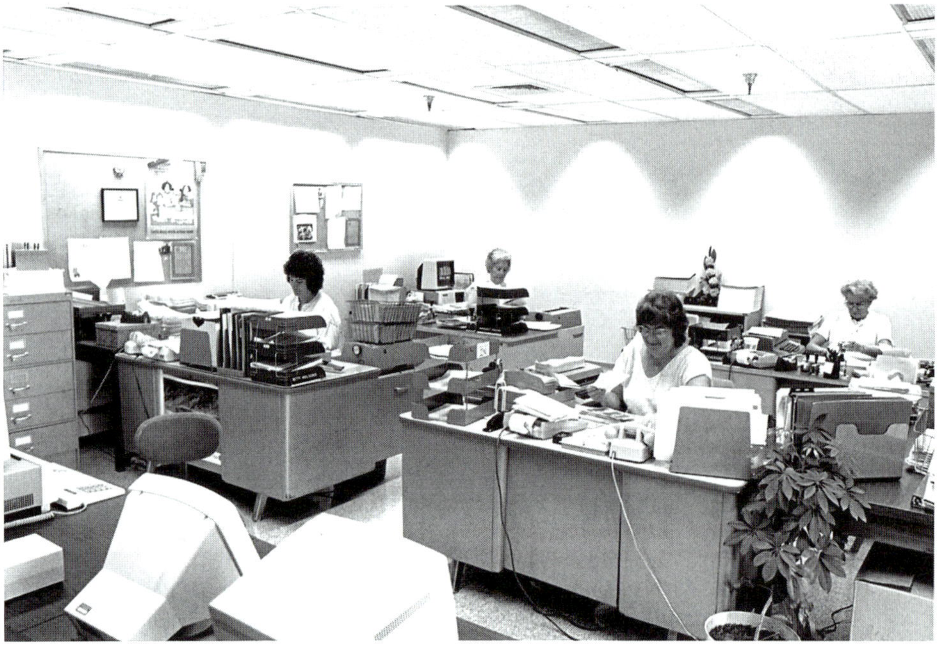

FIGURE 3— Office Workers Circa 1980s

Note. Open office plans were cited as having a strong potential for sick building syndrome. Note the lack of windows.
Source. Missouri Department of Conservation Photograph Collection. Courtesy of Missouri State Archives. Image Number: MDC_15-2524. Used with permission of Wikimedia under a Creative Commons license.

struggled to measure exposures and resigned themselves to recommending enhanced ventilation. It was only after decades of agitation by feminist activists that occupational health experts addressed toxic indoor chemicals. Ventilation was only one component in a matrix of historical forces: working conditions and gendered assumptions that cast female office workers as hypochondriacs shaped the intersection between air quality and chemical exposure.[42]

CONCLUSIONS

The pursuit of ventilation reinforces central questions of responsibility: who is responsible for health? What is the role of individual responsibility and of collective action? How does ventilation operate alongside other environmental and health interventions? The unregulated answers to these questions have underpinned radically uneven distributions of care. Although concerns over indoor air quality are old problems, the checkered history of ventilation reveals that any attempt to improve indoor air quality must consider its entanglement with social and environmental inequalities. Since ventilation emerged as a public health concern in the 18th century, attempts to improve air quality have had to contend with political and economic structures that have relegated poorer people to crowded and polluted neighborhoods, workplaces, and institutions.

COVID-19 brought these environmental and social inequalities into stark relief, as, despite considerable investment in ventilation and vaccination, the poor and incarcerated continued to suffer disproportionate rates of death and infection. A June 2022 article in the *Sacramento Bee* noted that despite separate wards, mandatory masking, and an 81% vaccination rate, nearly 75 000 incarcerated persons and 42 000 staff in California prisons had tested positive for COVID-19.[43] Incarcerated people are also more susceptible to injury and death from climate-driven extreme temperatures, and heat index temperatures have been recorded at higher than 150°F inside prisons.[44]

Whereas institutions like prisons remain inadequately regulated, there have been positive steps toward improving ventilation in schools. But despite the Biden administration's efforts at making funding and guidance available to school officials, much remains to be done. As reported in a recent article in the *New York Times*, no senior officials have been appointed to oversee the clean air initiative or help ensure that funds are spent effectively. The result is that many schools that would benefit are uncertain how to apply the funding or remain unaware that it exists.[45]

Ventilation has been stalked by inequity since its earliest incarnations as a public health strategy. One of Chadwick's most enduring and flawed legacies is the isolation of ventilation from other mandated environmental, economic, and political efforts. Today, as COVID-19 has reinvigorated concerns over air quality, we cannot continue to regard ventilation as a stand-alone intervention relying on individual responsibility. Virchow and Engels knew that air quality could not be understood apart from social inequalities. We, too, should recognize that improving ventilation is a political project that operates alongside and in other economic and environmental determinants of health. AJPH

ABOUT THE AUTHORS

Elaine LaFay is with the History Department, Rutgers University, New Brunswick, NJ. Paul E. Sampson is with the History Department, University of Scranton, Scranton, PA.

CORRESPONDENCE

Correspondence should be sent to Paul E. Sampson, 800 Linden Ave, Scranton, PA 18510 (e-mail: paul.sampson@scranton.edu). Reprints can be ordered at https://www.ajph.org by clicking the "Reprints" link.

PUBLICATION INFORMATION

Full Citation: LaFay E, Sampson P. Ventilation and public health: a fraught history. *Am J Public Health*. 2024;114(8):798–804.

Acceptance Date: March 22, 2024.

DOI: https://doi.org/10.2105/AJPH.2024.307670

CONTRIBUTORS

The authors conceptualized and wrote this essay collectively.

ACKNOWLEDGMENTS

Research for this article was partially supported by the Slattery Center for the Humanities, University of Scranton.

CONFLICTS OF INTEREST

The authors certify that they have no affiliations with or involvement in any organization or entity with any financial or nonfinancial interest in the subject matter or materials discussed in this article.

ENDNOTES

1. A. Mandavilli, "COVID Closed the Nations' Schools. Cleaner Air Can Keep Them Open," *New York Times*, August 27, 2023; Ladyzhets, "Your Kid's School Needs Better Ventilation to Help Keep COVID-19 in Check," *Time Magazine*, August 16, 2022; W. A. Haseltine, "How Enhanced Ventilation and Air Filtration Can Fight COVID-19," *Forbes*, October 21, 2022; T. Lewis and T. Bose, "How to Improve Indoor Air Quality," *Scientific American*, August 29, 2022; J. G. Allen, "Designing Buildings That Are Both Well-Ventilated and Green," *Harvard Business Review*, January 9, 2023.
2. Anon, "Fresh Thinking About Fresh Air," *The Economist*, May 29, 2021, 11.
3. The first edition appeared in 2020. A second edition with a revised title and a new chapter on the COVID-19 pandemic was published in 2022: J. G. Allen, J. D. Macomber, *Healthy Buildings: How Indoor Spaces Can Make You Sick—or Keep You Well*, 2nd ed. (Cambridge, MA: Harvard University Press, 2022), xii.
4. US Environmental Protection Agency, "Clean Air in Buildings Challenge," March 2022, https://www.epa.gov/system/files/documents/2022-03/508-cleanairbuildings_factsheet_v5_508.pdf (accessed May 14, 2024).
5. White House Office of Science and Technology Policy, "Virtual Event Transcript. Let's Clear the Air: An OSTP Discussion on COVID and Clean Indoor Air," March 29, 2022, https://www.whitehouse.gov/wp-content/uploads/2022/04/03-2022-Transcript-Lets-Clear-the-Air-on-COVID-

An-OSTP-Discussion-on-Clean-Indoor-Air.pdf (accessed May 14, 2024).

6. Anon., "Fresh Thinking About Fresh Air," 11.
7. The new London sewer embankments, for example, cost more than £2.4 million in 1869 (more than £234 million when adjusted for inflation). See S. Halliday, *The Great Stink of London* (Phoenix Mill, UK: Sutton Publishing, 2001), 148; "Inflation Calculator," Bank of England, August 16, 2023, https://www.bankofengland.co.uk/monetary-policy/inflation/inflation-calculator (accessed May 14, 2024).
8. C. Hamlin, "The 'Necessaries of Life' in British Political Medicine, 1750–1850," *Journal of Consumer Policy* 29 (2006): 373–396. https://doi.org/10.1007/s10603-006-9015-0
9. M. L. Bell, D. L. Davis, and T. Fletcher, "A Retrospective Assessment of Mortality From the London Smog Episode of 1952: The Role of Influenza and Pollution," *Environmental Health Perspectives* 112, no. 1 (2004): 6–8. https://doi.org/10.1289/ehp.6539
10. K. M. Schlichting and M. A. Kiechle, "Invisible Inequalities: Persistent Health Threats in the Urban Built Environment," *Journal of the History of Environment and Society* 5 (2020): 160. https://doi.org/10.1484/J.JHES.5.122472
11. A. Wear, "Place, Health and Disease: The Airs, Waters, Places Tradition in Early Modern England and North America," *Journal of Medieval and Early Modern Studies* 38, no. 3 (2008): 443–465. https://doi.org/10.1215/10829636-2008-003. See also C. E. Rosenberg, "Epilogue: Airs, Waters, Places. A Status Report," *Bulletin of the History of Medicine* 86, no. 4 (2012): 661–670. https://doi.org/10.1353/bhm.2012.0082; Indra Kagis McEwan has argued that Vitruvius's ambition to provide a "corpus" of architecture was a direct reference to how he believed the body should relate to the built environment. I. K. McEwan, *Vitruvius: Writing the Body of Architecture* (Cambridge, MA: MIT Press, 2003), 1–13.
12. J. Arbuthnot, *An Essay Concerning the Effects of Air on Human Bodies* (London, UK: J. Tonson, 1733), 148.
13. See, e.g., C. M. Cipolla, *Miasmas and Disease: Public Health and the Environment in the Pre-Industrial Age* (New Haven, CT: Yale University Press, 1992).
14. Typhus is a lice-borne disease, but early modern doctors were convinced that its transmission was airborne. See C. M. Blakley, "Ship Fever, Confinement, and the Racialization of Disease," *Studies in the History and Philosophy of Science* 95 (October 2022): 96–103. https://doi.org/10.1016/j.shpsa.2022.07.008; See P. E. Sampson, "'The Lungs of a Ship': Ventilation, Acclimatization, and the Maritime Environment, 1740–1800," *History of Science* 61, no. 2 (2023): 214–235. https://doi.org/10.1177/00732753211046449
15. S. Hales, *A Description of Ventilators* (London, UK: W. Innys, 1743) vi, 38.
16. H. Ellis, "A Letter to the Rev. Dr. Hales from Captain Henry Ellis," *Philosophical Transactions* 47 (1752): 213.
17. H. Ellis quoted in Stephen Hales, "An Account of the Great Benefit of Ventilators," *Philosophical Transactions* 49 (1755): 337.
18. M. Rediker, *The Slave Ship: A Human History* (London, UK: John Murray, 2007), 5; R. H. Steckel and R. A. Jensen, "Determinants of Slave and Crew Mortality in the Atlantic Slave Trade" (Cambridge, MA: National Bureau of Economic Research, 1985), 6. NBER working paper 1540.
19. W. Elford, *Remarks on the Slave Trade* (Samuel Wood, 1788); Marcus Rediker, *The Slave Ship: A Human History* (New York, NY: John Murray, 2007), 311–314.
20. Act for Preserving the Health of Prisoners in Gaol and Preventing the Gaol Distemper, 1774, 14 Geo. III, c. 59.
21. Enslaved people on antebellum plantations adopted similar strategies of managing ventilation on their own terms. E. LaFay, "'The Wind Can Blow Through and Through': Ventilation, Public Health, and the Regulation of Fresh Air on Antebellum Southern Plantations," in *Atlantic Environments and the American South: An Anthology*, ed. T. B. Earle and D. A. Johnson II (Athens, GA: University of Georgia Press, 2020), 38–62.
22. R. Evans, *The Fabrication of Virtue* (London, UK: Cambridge University Press, 1982), 162–163.
23. M. Ignatieff, *A Just Measure of Pain* (London, UK: Penguin, 1978), 3–14.
24. G. Blane, "Letter to John Hippisley," in *Observations on the Diseases of Seamen* (London, UK: Murray and Highley, 1799), 614–615.
25. A Physician of Philadelphia, *The Home Book of Health and Medicine: A Popular Treatise on the Means of Avoiding and Curing Diseases, and of Preserving the Health and Vigour of the Body to the Latest Period* (Philadelphia, PA: Key & Biddle, 1835), 102.
26. P. Bingham, N. Q. Verlander, and M. J. Cheal, "John Snow, William Farr and the 1849 Outbreak of Cholera That Affected London: A Reworking of the Data Highlights the Importance of the Water Supply," *Public Health* 118, no. 6 (2004): 387–394. https://doi.org/10.1016/j.puhe.2004.05.007
27. For a discussion of vitiated air, see M. Kiechle, *Smell Detectives* (Seattle, WA: University of Washington Press, 2017), 27.
28. F. Nightingale, *Notes on Nursing: What It Is, and What It Is Not* (New York, NY: D. Appleton and Company, 1860), 12.
29. See S. Halliday, "Death and Miasma in Victorian London: An Obstinate Belief," *British Medical Journal* 323, no. 7327 (2001): 1469–1471. https://doi.org/10.1136/bmj.323.7327.1469
30. E. Chadwick, *Report from the Poor Law Commissioners on an Inquiry Into the Sanitary Conditions of the Labouring Population of Great Britain* (London, UK: W. Clowes and Sons, 1842), 369.
31. On commodification of air, see M. Thébaud-Sorger, "Capturing the Invisible: Heat, Steam and Gases in France and Great Britain, 1750–1800," in *Compound Histories: Materials, Governance and Production, 1760–1840*, ed. L. Roberts and S. Werrett (Leiden, Netherlands: Brill, 2018), 85–105.
32. New York Association for Improving the Condition of the Poor, *First Report of a Committee on the Sanitary Condition of the Laboring Classes in the City of New-York, With Remedial Suggestions* (New York, NY: John F. Trow & Co., 1853), 10.
33. Ibid., 4.
34. K. M. Schlichting and M. A. Kiechle, "Invisible Inequalities," 162–164.
35. R. Virchow, "On Famine Fever and Some of the Other Cognate Forms of Typhus: A Lecture Held for the Benefit of the Sufferers in East Prussia, February 9, 1868" (London, UK: Williams and Norgate, 1868), 46.
36. F. Engels, *The Condition of the Working Class in England in 1844* (London, UK: Swan Sonnenschein & Co., 1892), 158.
37. C. Hamlin, *Public Health and Social Justice in the Age of Chadwick: Britain, 1800–1854* (Cambridge, UK: Cambridge University Press, 1998).
38. A. Rabinbach, *The Human Motor: Energy, Fatigue, and the Origins of Modernity* (Berkeley, CA: University of California Press, 1992), 2.
39. New York State Commission on Ventilation, *Ventilation: Report of the New York State Commission on Ventilation* (New York, NY: E. P. Dutton, 1923).
40. For example, F. Taylor, *The Principles of Scientific Management* (New York, NY: Harper & Brothers Publishers, 1915); P. Drinker, "Laboratories of Ventilation and Illumination, Harvard School of Public Health, Boston," *Journal of Industrial Hygiene* 6, no. 1 (1924): 57–66. On Taylorism, see M. Banta, *Taylored Lives: Narrative Productions in the Age of Taylor, Veblen, and Ford* (Chicago, IL: University of Chicago Press, 1992).
41. M. Murphy, *Sick Building Syndrome and the Problem of Uncertainty* (Durham, NC: Duke University Press, 2006).
42. Ibid.
43. M. McGough, "More COVID-19 Outbreaks Reported at California Prisons, Among Inmates and Staff," *Sacramento Bee*, June 1, 2022, https://www.sacbee.com/news/coronavirus/article262021837.html (accessed May 14, 2024).
44. D. W. E. Holt, *Heat in US Prisons and Jails: Corrections and the Challenge of Climate Change*, https://bit.ly/4bjJflr (accessed May 14, 2024). https://doi.org/10.2139/ssrn.2667260
45. A. Mandavilli, "COVID Closed the Nations' Schools. Cleaner Air Can Keep Them Open," *New York Times*, August 27, 2023, https://www.nytimes.com/2023/08/27/health/schools-indoor-air-covid.html?searchResultPosition=2 (accessed May 14, 2024).

Examining the Impact of Minimum Handgun Purchase Age and Background Check Legislation on Young Adult Suicide in the United States, 1991–2020

Emma E. Fridel, PhD, Gregory M. Zimmerman, PhD, and Shayna R. Arrigo, BA

See also Peck, p. 766.

Objectives. To examine the independent and joint effects of state legislation on minimum age for purchasing handguns and background checks on the suicide of young adults aged 18 to 20 years.

Methods. We used negative binomial regressions with fixed effects for year and generalized estimating equations for state to estimate the effects of state legislation on annual counts of firearm, nonfirearm, and total young adult suicides in all 50 US states from 1991 to 2020.

Results. Minimum age laws decreased the incidence rate of firearm suicide among young adults, an effect that was amplified in states with permit to purchase laws; there was no effect on the nonfirearm or total suicide rate. Permit to purchase laws significantly decreased the young adult firearm suicide incidence rate by 39% (incidence rate ratio [IRR] = 0.61; 95% confidence interval [CI] = 0.51, 0.74) and the overall suicide incidence rate by 14% (IRR = 0.86; 95% CI = 0.75, 0.99), with no effect on the nonfirearm suicide rate.

Conclusions. Permit to purchase laws are a more promising avenue for reducing young adult suicides than are age-based restrictions. (*Am J Public Health*. 2024;114(8):805–813. https://doi.org/10.2105/AJPH.2024.307689)

AJPH August 2024, Vol. 114, No. 8

In 2020, suicide was the third leading cause of death among persons aged 18 to 20 years in the United States, accounting for 1750 deaths.[1] Firearms were used in approximately half of these incidents and surpassed motor vehicles as the leading mechanism of death in 2017.[2] Following several high-profile shootings, public and political support for restricting access to firearms for this vulnerable population surged, with 79% of people in the United States supporting raising the minimum age to purchase guns to 21 years.[3]

Federal law has mandated a minimum age of 21 years to purchase handguns and 18 years to purchase long guns from licensed dealers since 1968 (18 USC § 922(b)(1), (c)(1)) and a minimum age of 18 years to purchase handguns from private sellers since 1994 (18 USC § 922(x)(1), (5)). Federal law also prohibits the possession of handguns and handgun ammunition by persons younger than 18 years. Currently, there are no federal restrictions for purchasing long guns from private sellers or possessing long guns or ammunition. Corresponding with research that the human brain continues to develop impulse control into the mid-20s,[4] 17 states prohibited handgun purchases from private sellers for individuals younger than 21 years as of 2020, 8 extended this restriction to handgun possession, and 8 included handgun ammunition.

Although previous work has examined the impact of age-based gun control legislation on firearm fatalities of children younger than 18 years, less is known about policies targeting young adults aged 18 to 20 years.[5] This is surprising, as young adults have greater access to firearms and are at higher risk for violence. The handful of studies in this line of inquiry examined the impact of raising the federal minimum purchasing age from 18 to 21 years, producing mixed findings. Some studies found no evidence of a protective effect on suicide,[6–9] whereas others suggested that state minimum age laws are associated with approximately 2 fewer suicides per 100 000 young adults.[10,11]

These conflicting findings may be explained in part by the failure to consider the mechanism by which the law works. As Rowhani-Rahbar et al. note,

> Changes in firearm policies do not occur in a vacuum. . .. They may collectively or synergistically compound that risk [firearm suicide] through interacting with each other and with other existing policies.[12(p2)]

State minimum age restrictions specifically target purchases from private sellers, as federal law already prohibits individuals younger than 21 years from purchasing handguns from licensed dealers. As private sellers are not required to conduct background checks under federal law (i.e., the "gun show loophole"), states must enforce minimum age restrictions by mandating universal background checks at point of sale or through a permit to purchase (PTP). Although previous studies often controlled for universal background checks or PTP laws, none has examined whether the impact of state minimum age laws on the incidence of young adult suicide depends on background check legislation.

Heeding the call to pursue mechanistic explanations,[12] we examined the independent and joint impacts of state minimum age and background check legislation on the incidence rate of suicide among young adults. Using cross-sectional panel models with fixed effects and generalized estimating equations, we examined the direct effect of state minimum age laws on young adult suicides and the moderating role of universal background check and PTP laws on the effect of state minimum age laws as an enforcement mechanism.

METHODS

We used a quasiexperimental design to take advantage of changes in state minimum age and background check laws over time. Using cross-sectional panel models, we explored the relationship between these laws and suicides (by firearm, by other methods, and in total) among persons aged 18 to 20 years in the 50 US states from 1991 to 2020. We obtained data on suicide by age and method of death from the Centers for Disease Control and Prevention's Web-based Injury Statistics Query and Reporting System (WISQARS). WISQARS is an ideal suicide data source, as it extracts information from standardized death certificates directly and has a 99% reporting rate across the United States.[2]

Information on firearm legislation over time was provided by the State Firearm Laws Database, which used Thomson Reuters Westlaw to track the presence or absence of more than 100 firearm provisions by state since 1991.[13] We coded all laws based on their effective date. We appended annual state-level data on 12 control variables from multiple sources, including the US Census Bureau, Uniform Crime Reports, the National Vital Statistics System, the Bureau of Justice Statistics, the National Institute of Alcoholism and Alcohol Abuse, and the Centers for Medicare & Medicaid Services. Study variables and their data sources are described in Appendix Table A (available as a supplement to the online version of this article at http://www.ajph.org).

Measures

Outcome and key independent variables. Outcomes included the annual state count of suicides by firearm (*ICD-10* [*International Classification of Diseases, 10th Revision* (Geneva, Switzerland: World Health Organization); 1992] codes X72-X74), other methods (*ICD-10* codes X60-X71, X75-X84), and in total (*ICD-10* codes X60-X84) of persons aged 18 to 20 years. We measured suicide as a count because of its relative rarity and the small population of interest.

We measured state firearm legislation with a series of binary variables (1 = law is in effect; 0 = law is not in effect). We lagged all laws by 1 year to ensure that they applied to the suicide decedent at time of death. Key provisions of interest included a minimum age of 21 years to purchase a handgun (10 states in 1991; 17 states in 2020), a minimum age of 21 years to purchase handgun ammunition (1 state in 1991; 8 states in 2020), permit required to purchase or carry all firearms (5 states in 1991; 7 states in 2020), and background checks required at point-of-sale for all firearms (i.e., universal background checks; 2 states in 1991; 12 states in 2020).[13] We included the total number of firearm laws (standardized) as a general measure of gun control in the state. The year of implementation for the 4 laws of interest is shown by state in Table 1.

Control variables. The analysis controlled for concentrated disadvantage, racial/ethnic heterogeneity, violent and property crime rates, incarceration

AJPH August 2024, Vol. 114, No. 8

TABLE 1— Year of Implementation for State Minimum Age and Background Check Laws for Firearm Purchase: United States, 1991–2020

State	Minimum Age of 21 y to Purchase Handgun	Minimum Age of 21 y to Purchase Handgun Ammunition	Permit to Purchase for All Firearms	Point-of-Sale Background Checks for All Firearms
California	1985	1997	2015	1991
Colorado	...	...	...	2013
Connecticut	1994	2013	2014	1999
Delaware	1987	...	...	2013
Florida	2018	...	...	...
Georgia	Pre-1976–1993	...	...	...
Hawaii	1994	...	1981	...
Illinois	...	...	Pre-1976	...
Iowa	1979	1978	...	...
Maryland	1996	1996	...	...
Massachusetts	1998	1998	Pre-1976	...
Missouri	1981–2006	...	...	...
Nebraska	1991	...	...	...
Nevada	...	...	...	2017
New Jersey	2001	2008	Pre-1976	...
New Mexico	...	...	...	2019
New York	2000	2000	...	2013
Ohio	Pre-1976	...	...	...
Oregon	...	...	...	2015
Rhode Island	Pre-1976	...	1990	1990
South Carolina	Pre-1976–2007	...	...	...
Vermont	2018	...	...	2018
Virginia	...	...	...	2020
Washington	Pre-1976–1993, 2019 to present	...	...	2014
West Virginia	2010	2010	...	...
Wyoming	2010	...	...	...

Note. States not shown did not implement or change these 4 laws between 1976 and 2020.
Source. State Firearms Laws Database.

rates, high school graduation rates, per capita alcohol consumption, hospital expenditures per capita, percentage of the population that is male, and census region (South vs Northeast, West, or Midwest). We measured household gun ownership using a restricted version of the most common and reliable proxy: the proportion of suicides committed with firearms (excluding persons aged 18–20 years).[14] We also controlled for the divorce rate based on research demonstrating that parental divorce increases the odds of adult children attempting suicide.[15] Finally, we included the suicide rate per 100 000 for persons aged 21 to 23 years to control for unobserved factors that influence suicide rates among similarly aged persons across space and time, such as social norms.[6]

Analytical Strategy

Using cross-sectional panel models with negative binomial regression, we estimated changes in the effects of state minimum age and background check laws over time on the incidence rate of suicides of young adults aged 18 to 20 years. This approach is appropriate for count data that are overdispersed.[6] In comparison with alternate strategies such as the synthetic control method, it also can estimate interactive effects of 2 policy interventions implemented at different points in time, the focus of this study.[12] We included the natural logarithm of the total population aged 18 to 20 years as an offset. We imputed missing data on the divorce, incarceration, and high school graduation rate in Stata version 15 (StataCorp LP, College Station, TX) with chained equations. We standardized all continuous variables.

The model accounted for clustering by year and state. We included year fixed effects to purge the model of cross-sectional bias. Following previous work,[6,16] we used generalized estimating equations (GEEs) to control for clustering in states over time. A population-averaged or marginal approach, GEEs treat dependence as a nuisance feature of the data.[17] As GEEs require no assumptions about the distribution, they are relatively unaffected by misspecification of the working correlation matrix. We used an exchangeable (compound symmetry) working correlation matrix and robust (Huber-White sandwich estimators) SEs to produce consistent point estimates and SEs even if the working correlation matrix was misspecified.[17] The semiparametric nature of GEEs lowers the model power, indicating that the results are conservative.

RESULTS

Firearm laws focused on young adults have become more prevalent over the past 30 years (Table 1). In 1991, 10 states required a minimum age of 21 years to purchase a handgun. By 2020, 17 states had raised the federal minimum handgun purchasing age, with 14 states changing their policies over the study period (including 10 adopting, 3 repealing, and 1 repealing and readopting). Although only 1 state (Iowa) extended such restrictions to purchasing handgun ammunition in 1991, the number has grown to 8 states as of 2020. The background check laws required to enforce these age-based restrictions for purchases from private sellers have also become more common. The number of states requiring a PTP for all firearms increased from 5 in 1991 to 7 by 2020. The change was more dramatic for point-of-sale background checks for all firearms, increasing from 2 states at the beginning of the study period to 12 by 2020. No states repealed existing background check legislation during the study period.

Figure 1 shows the age-adjusted national suicide rate for persons aged 18 to 20 years per 100 000 population from 1991 to 2020 (Appendix Table D, available as a supplement to the online version of this article at http://www.ajph.org). The young adult suicide rate decreased throughout the late 1990s and early 2000s, from 14.06 in 1994 to 9.93 in 2007; suicides involving firearms exhibited a similar pattern, decreasing from a rate of 9.55 in 1994 to 4.12 in 2010. Following these historic decreases, the young adult suicide rate surged in the early 2010s, exceeding the record levels of the 1990s with a high of 14.95 in 2017. The firearm suicide rate increased modestly over the same period,

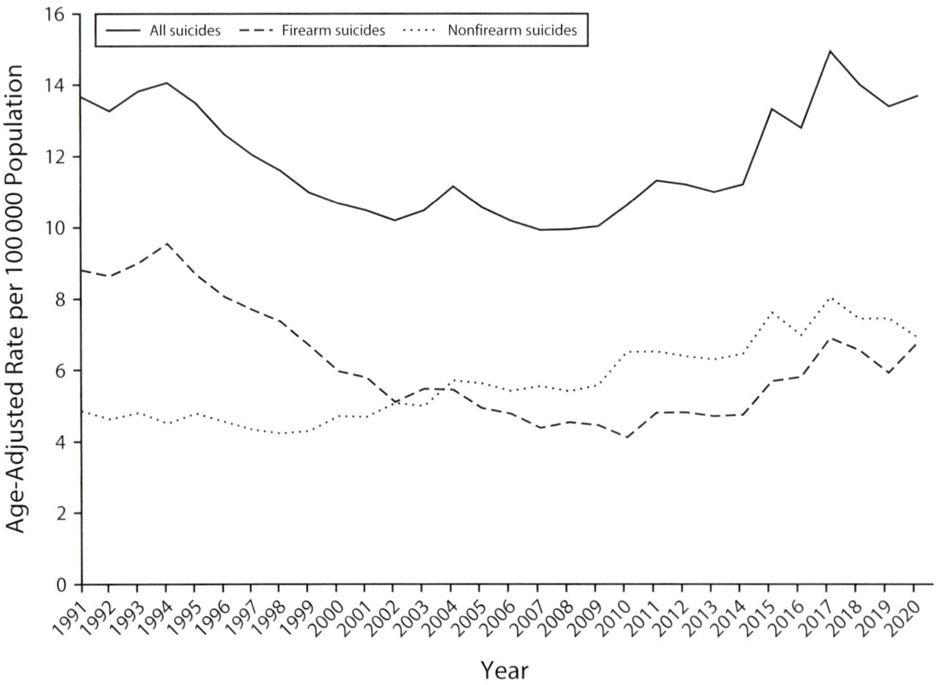

FIGURE 1— **Age-Adjusted National Suicide Rate for Young Adults Aged 18 to 20 Years: United States, 1991–2020**

peaking at a rate of 6.9 in 2017. By contrast, the nonfirearm suicide rate fluctuated between 4.23 and 5.08 in the early 1990s and 2000s, first exceeding the firearm rate in 2004 and then steadily increasing to a high of 8.05 in 2017. In 2020, suicide rates by method were approximately equal.

Minimum Purchasing Age and Young Adult Suicides

Effects on incidence rate of young adult suicides. Table 2 presents the results of the population-averaged negative binomial regressions on suicide by firearm, other methods, and in total. Standardized regression coefficients in the form of incidence rate ratios (IRRs) and 95% confidence intervals (CIs) are presented to facilitate interpretation. IRRs indicate the percentage increase or decrease in the outcome incidence rate for every SD increase in the predictor ([IRR – 1] × 100%).

As shown in the base models, state laws increasing the minimum purchase age for handguns to 21 years were associated with a 12% reduction in the incidence of firearm suicide among those aged 18 to 20 years (IRR = 0.88; 95% CI = 0.79, 0.98) yet had no significant impact on nonfirearm suicide (IRR = 1.00; 95% CI = 0.93, 1.08) or the overall suicide rate (IRR = 0.98; 95% CI = 0.91, 1.06). These results are consistent with the work of Webster et al.,[6] in both significance and magnitude. By contrast, state PTP laws significantly decreased the young adult firearm suicide incidence rate by 39% (IRR = 0.61; 95% CI = 0.51, 0.74) and the overall suicide incidence rate by 14% (IRR = 0.86; 95% CI = 0.75, 0.99), with no significant impact on nonfirearm suicides (IRR = 1.00;

TABLE 2— Population-Averaged Negative Binomial Regressions on Young Adult Firearm, Nonfirearm, and Total Suicides in the 50 US States, 1991–2020

Predictors	Base Model, IRR (95% CI)			Interaction Model, IRR (95% CI)		
	Firearms Suicide	Nonfirearms Suicide	Total Suicide	Firearms Suicide	Nonfirearms Suicide	Total Suicide
Gun control legislation						
Aged 21 y to purchase handguns	0.88 (0.79, 0.98)	1.00 (0.93, 1.08)	0.98 (0.91, 1.06)	0.92 (0.84, 1.01)	1.03 (0.95, 1.12)	0.98 (0.91, 1.06)
Permit to purchase	0.61 (0.51, 0.74)	1.00 (0.85, 1.16)	0.86 (0.75, 0.99)	0.77 (0.69, 0.87)	1.12 (0.87, 1.42)	0.84 (0.71, 0.99)
Purchase age x permit to purchase	...	...	...	0.72 (0.59, 0.88)	0.87 (0.71, 1.07)	1.03 (0.89, 1.20)
Aged 21 y to purchase handgun ammunition	0.97 (0.81, 1.15)	0.90 (0.77, 1.05)	0.94 (0.83, 1.07)	1.03 (0.87, 1.21)	0.91 (0.79, 1.06)	0.94 (0.83, 1.07)
Point-of-sale background checks	0.97 (0.87, 1.08)	0.97 (0.87, 1.09)	0.98 (0.91, 1.07)	0.99 (0.89, 1.10)	0.97 (0.87, 1.09)	0.98 (0.91, 1.07)
Total number of laws (standardized)	0.90 (0.83, 0.99)	1.02 (0.92, 1.14)	0.97 (0.89, 1.05)	0.88 (0.81, 0.96)	1.01 (0.91, 1.13)	0.97 (0.90, 1.05)
Sociodemographic controls						
Gun ownership	1.23 (1.14, 1.32)	1.03 (0.93, 1.14)	1.11 (1.05, 1.17)	1.23 (1.15, 1.32)	1.03 (0.93, 1.14)	1.11 (1.05, 1.17)
Concentrated disadvantage	1.01 (0.97, 1.05)	0.97 (0.93, 1.01)	0.99 (0.96, 1.02)	1.01 (0.98, 1.05)	0.97 (0.93, 1.01)	0.99 (0.96, 1.02)
Racial/ethnic heterogeneity	0.95 (0.86, 1.04)	1.08 (1.00, 1.17)	1.03 (0.96, 1.11)	0.95 (0.87, 1.04)	1.08 (1.00, 1.17)	1.03 (0.96, 1.11)
Violent crime rate	1.05 (1.00, 1.10)	0.99 (0.94, 1.04)	1.00 (0.96, 1.03)	1.05 (1.00, 1.09)	0.99 (0.94, 1.04)	1.00 (0.97, 1.03)
Property crime rate	1.07 (1.03, 1.12)	1.01 (0.96, 1.07)	1.02 (0.99, 1.06)	1.08 (1.03, 1.12)	1.01 (0.96, 1.07)	1.02 (0.99, 1.06)
Divorce rate	1.02 (0.98, 1.06)	1.00 (0.95, 1.05)	1.04 (0.99, 1.08)	1.02 (0.99, 1.06)	1.00 (0.95, 1.06)	1.04 (0.99, 1.08)
Incarceration rate	1.01 (0.95, 1.07)	1.00 (0.95, 1.05)	0.98 (0.94, 1.03)	1.00 (0.94, 1.06)	0.99 (0.94, 1.05)	0.98 (0.94, 1.03)
High school graduation rate	1.02 (0.99, 1.06)	1.04 (1.00, 1.08)	1.02 (1.00, 1.05)	1.02 (0.99, 1.05)	1.04 (1.00, 1.08)	1.02 (1.00, 1.05)
Alcohol consumption per capita	0.98 (0.95, 1.00)	0.95 (0.91, 1.00)	0.98 (0.95, 1.02)	0.98 (0.96, 1.00)	0.96 (0.91, 1.00)	0.98 (0.95, 1.02)
Hospital expenditures	1.08 (1.03, 1.12)	1.04 (0.97, 1.11)	1.04 (0.99, 1.09)	1.07 (1.03, 1.11)	1.03 (0.97, 1.11)	1.04 (0.99, 1.09)
Percentage male	1.21 (1.14, 1.29)	1.11 (1.03, 1.20)	1.14 (1.08, 1.20)	1.21 (1.15, 1.28)	1.11 (1.02, 1.20)	1.14 (1.08, 1.20)
Suicide rate for persons aged 21–23 y	1.07 (1.02, 1.12)	1.08 (1.04, 1.12)	1.06 (1.03, 1.10)	1.08 (1.03, 1.13)	1.08 (1.04, 1.12)	1.06 (1.03, 1.10)
US Southern region[a]	0.92 (0.83, 1.03)	0.75 (0.66, 0.85)	0.86 (0.78, 0.94)	0.93 (0.85, 1.03)	0.75 (0.66, 0.85)	0.86 (0.78, 0.94)

Note. CI = confidence interval; IRR = incidence rate ratio. Fixed effects for year not shown.
[a]Southern US region includes the following states: AL, AR, DE, FL, GA, KY, LA, MD, MS, NC, OK, SC, TN, TX, VA, and WV.

95% CI = 0.85, 1.16). State laws raising the minimum age to purchase handgun ammunition and mandating point-of-sale background checks did not have a significant impact on any of the outcomes. The findings were largely unchanged when we included state laws raising the minimum age to possess a handgun to 21 years in addition to or instead of purchasing regulations.

Interaction with background check legislation. As shown in the interaction models in Table 2, the effect of state laws raising the minimum purchase age for handguns on young adult suicide was moderated by PTP laws. For a state with minimum age restrictions, implementing PTP laws reduced the IRR, representing the effect of minimum age laws, by 0.28 (IRR = 0.72; 95% CI = 0.59, 0.88). In other words, although minimum age restrictions have no effect on firearm suicide rates in states without PTP laws (IRR = 0.92; 95% CI = 0.84, 1.01), they decrease the firearm suicide incidence rate by 33% in states with PTP laws (IRR = 0.67; 95% CI = 0.54, 0.81; results calculated in models not shown here). These results suggest that the protective effects of minimum age laws are contingent on PTP laws. The interaction effect was not significant in the nonfirearm and total suicide rate models.

Furthermore, there were no significant interaction effects between ammunition regulations and PTP laws, whereas interaction effects involving point-of-sale background checks varied depending on model specification (see Appendix Table B [available as a supplement to the online version of this article at http://www.ajph.org] for point estimates of PTP and universal background check interactions with the 3 age-based restrictions).

The study findings are visualized in Figure 2, which shows the predicted number of firearm, nonfirearm, and total suicides among young adults aged 18 to 20 years by state firearm legislation. The average state that had not adopted either type of law had approximately 31 young adult suicides in an average year, 16 of which involved firearms. By comparison, states with minimum purchasing age laws alone had 2 fewer firearm suicides, whereas those with only PTP laws had a reduction 3 times as large, or 6 prevented deaths. States that passed both laws had the fewest number of firearm suicides, with more than 1 additional death prevented beyond the adoption of PTP laws alone.

By contrast, the average state had approximately 15 suicides by other methods, regardless of minimum purchasing age and PTP legislation. Because of relatively wide CIs for the predicted number of total suicides, it is unclear whether the reduction in firearm suicides in states with minimum purchasing age laws resulted in a net reduction

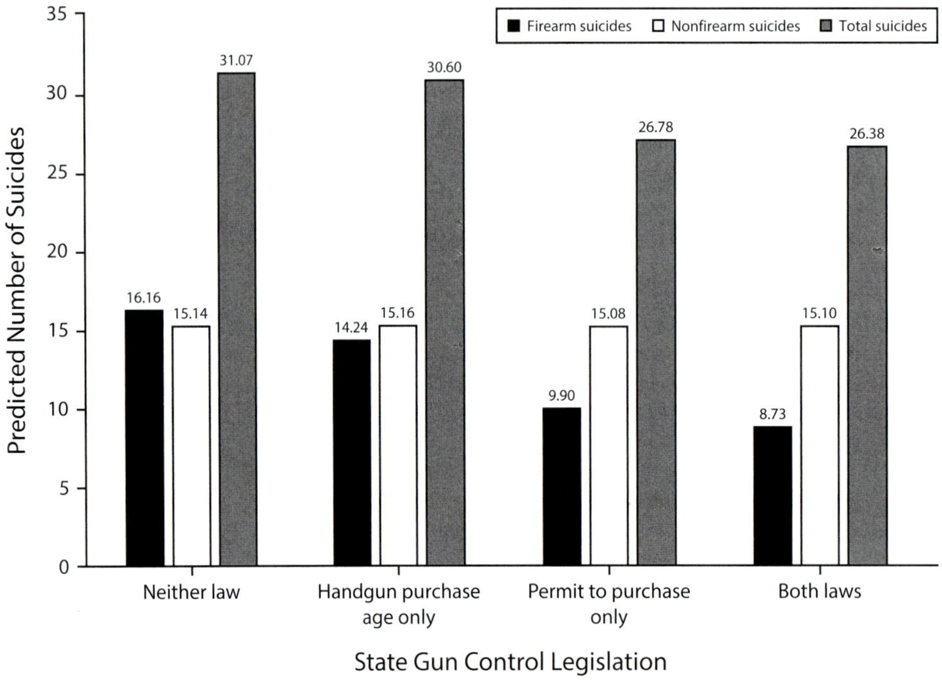

FIGURE 2— **Predicted Annual Number of Firearm, Nonfirearm, and Total Suicides for Young Adults Aged 18–20 Years by State Gun Control Legislation: United States, 1991–2020**

in the overall number of young adult suicides. States with PTP laws, however, had 4 fewer suicides (regardless of method) each year.

Sensitivity Analyses

We conducted various robustness checks to ensure the validity of the results. Findings remained substantively unchanged when

1. we employed Poisson regression with fixed effects for year and state instead of GEEs,[18]
2. we measured the outcome as a rate per 100 000 population and analyzed it with ordinary least squares regression,
3. we restricted the study timeframe to the period after the passage of federal legislation in 1994,
4. we restricted the study period to exclude 2020 because of the COVID-19 pandemic,
5. we substituted an alternate measure of gun ownership proposed by RAND,[19]
6. we excluded imputed variables (including the divorce, incarceration, and high school graduation rates),
7. we included only 1 gun control law in the model at a time, and
8. we added additional gun control laws, including a minimum age of 21 years to purchase long guns, mandatory waiting periods for all firearm purchases, prohibitions for persons involuntarily committed to outpatient facilities, "red flag" laws, child access prevention laws, and mandatory reporting of firearm loss or theft by all owners.

Across these different model specifications, point estimates for the effect of PTP laws ranged from an IRR of 0.55 (95% CI = 0.43, 0.71) to an IRR of 0.69 (95% CI = 0.57, 0.83) for firearm suicide and from an IRR of 0.83 (95% CI = 0.72, 0.95) to an IRR of 0.88 (95% CI = 0.76, 1.01) for total suicide; PTP laws did not affect nonfirearm suicide in any of the model specifications (Appendix Table C, available as a supplement to the online version of this article at http://www.ajph.org). Models changing the target population to a negative control group—persons aged 21 years and older—indicated that minimum age laws have no significant impact on the incidence rate of firearm, nonfirearm, or total suicides.

DISCUSSION

This study contributes to the literature on strategies to reduce young adult suicide by examining the effects of state minimum age laws to purchase handguns and their primary enforcement mechanism: background checks. Using data that span several decades, we are the first to our knowledge to report that the impact of state minimum handgun purchasing age laws on the incidence of young adult firearm suicide is contingent on state PTP legislation. Findings indicated that the average state that has not adopted either policy had approximately 16 young adult firearm suicides in an average year.

In comparison, states with minimum purchasing age laws alone had 14 firearm suicides, a figure reduced to fewer than 10 in states with both laws. However, it remains unclear whether the joint effects of state minimum age and PTP legislation extend to total suicides. Previous work has also reported inconsistent results when comparing disaggregated (firearm and nonfirearm) and total suicide models,[6] which may be an artifact of the rarity of the outcome, limited target population, and small effect size of the law.[20] For example, the proportion of young adult suicides involving firearms decreased from approximately two thirds to less than one half during the study period, reducing the intervention population size.

Therefore, it is possible that age-based restrictions for handguns have a significant yet small protective effect that the full model was unable to detect; alternatively, young adults may substitute handguns for other methods or long guns. For example, recent work suggests that one fourth of all suicides are committed with long guns,[21] a proportion that increases to 37% for individuals in the target age group (18–24 years).[22] Another explanation regards the ease with which young adults obtain guns from family members or friends. Indeed, three fourths of firearm suicide decedents younger than 21 years obtained the gun from someone else.[23]

By contrast, PTP laws reduced the incidence rate of firearm suicide by 39% and total suicide by 14% among young adults aged 18 to 20 years, with no significant change in nonfirearm suicide. The results thus contribute to the growing body of literature suggesting that PTP laws are effective in reducing suicide[24,25] and homicide.[26,27] Consistent with previous work, point-of-sale background checks did not appear to affect young adult suicide, either independently or in tandem with minimum age laws.[25,28]

Limitations

The findings are tempered by several limitations. Although more states have PTP or universal background check laws for handguns only, we were unable to disaggregate suicides by type of firearm (handgun or long gun), as

WISQARS classifies most firearm-related deaths as "other and unspecified" firearm because of the lack of specificity on death certificates.[29] Similarly, we were able to include minimum age laws for long gun purchasing only as a control variable because of the rarity and recency of these restrictions. Until 2017, Hawaii was the only state to raise the federal minimum purchasing age for long guns to 21 years. Future research is needed to examine the impact of weapon-specific minimum age and background check legislation, but the current lack of data poses significant challenges in this regard.

Public Health Implications

With these limitations in mind, the findings suggest that age-based handgun restrictions have a small if not negligible impact on young adult suicides, potentially because of means substitution, use of long guns, access to household firearms, or the fact that these restrictions relate only to the private sale of handguns (as federal law already prohibits the sale of handguns by dealers). Taken together, the results suggest that alternate laws designed to reduce firearm access in general—rather than for this age group in particular—may be more fruitful. Especially promising are PTP laws, which require individuals to apply for a firearm permit in person with a local or state law enforcement agency before purchase. The policies are often accompanied by fingerprint identification and an extended background check searching both state and federal records, increasing the likelihood that law enforcement will detect a prohibiting condition.

Although PTP laws affect individuals across the life-span, they may be especially effective for young adults. Interacting face-to-face with law enforcement during the permitting process likely discourages underage buyers and increases the perceived risks for straw purchasers. Similarly, licensing fees and mandatory firearm safety–training classes may be cost prohibitive for unemployed or in-school young adults. The increased scrutiny of PTP vetting procedures is also time consuming, reducing the potential for impulsive suicide attempts.[12,25] Indeed, approximately half of survivors of near-lethal suicide attempts deliberate for less than 10 minutes before acting,[30] and some previous work suggests that younger individuals are more likely to impulsively attempt suicide.[31] PTP laws may also indirectly prevent young adult suicide by reducing overall levels of gun ownership, making it more difficult to use the firearms of friends and family members.

Given that PTP laws vary across states in terms of their requirements, waiting periods, and permit duration, more research is needed to understand which provisions are effective in reducing suicide, for both young adults and the general population. Handgun permits are valid for only 10 days in Hawaii and Massachusetts, for example, yet licenses in Illinois do not expire for 10 years. Similarly, more work is needed to disentangle the effects of PTP laws and point-of-sale background checks on firearm violence, as many states have enacted both policies. Despite these gaps in the literature, PTP laws are critical for limiting access to lethal means for at-risk individuals, including young adults. The fact that more than three quarters of people in the United States support them makes licensing laws an evidence-based and politically feasible policy intervention for reducing firearm suicide.[32] AJPH

ABOUT THE AUTHORS

Emma E. Fridel and Shayna R. Arrigo are with the College of Criminology and Criminal Justice, Florida State University, Tallahassee. Gregory M. Zimmerman is with the School of Criminology and Criminal Justice, Northeastern University, Boston, MA.

CORRESPONDENCE

Correspondence should be sent to Emma E. Fridel, 408 Criminology and Criminal Justice Building, 112 South Copeland St, Florida State University, Tallahassee, FL 32304 (e-mail: efridel@fsu.edu). Reprints can be ordered at https://www.ajph.org by clicking the "Reprints" link.

PUBLICATION INFORMATION

Full Citation: Fridel EE, Zimmerman GM, Arrigo SR. Examining the impact of minimum handgun purchase age and background check legislation on young adult suicide in the United States, 1991–2020. *Am J Public Health*. 2024;114(8):805–813.

Acceptance Date: April 5, 2024.

DOI: https://doi.org/10.2105/AJPH.2024.307689

ORCID iD:

Emma E. Fridel https://orcid.org/0000-0001-9346-2156

CONTRIBUTORS

E. E. Fridel conceptualized the study, cleaned the data, conducted the analyses, and wrote the article. G. M. Zimmerman interpreted the analyses and wrote the article. S. R Arrigo obtained and cleaned the data. All authors critically reviewed and commented on the article.

CONFLICTS OF INTEREST

The authors have no conflicts of interest to disclose.

HUMAN PARTICIPANT PROTECTION

Institutional review board approval was not required for this study as it did not involve human participants and all data were from secondary sources.

REFERENCES

1. Centers for Disease Control and Prevention. Wide-ranging ONline Data for Epidemiologic Research: multiple cause of death data. 2023. Available at: https://wonder.cdc.gov/mcd.html. Accessed May 20, 2024.
2. Centers for Disease Control and Prevention. Web-based Injury Statistics Query and Reporting System: fatal injury data. 2023. Available at: https://www.cdc.gov/injury/wisqars/fatal/trends.html. Accessed May 20, 2024.
3. Pew Research Center. Gun violence widely viewed as a major—and growing—national problem. 2023. Available at: https://www.pewresearch.org/politics/2023/06/28/gun-violence-widely-viewed-as-a-major-and-growing-national-problem. Accessed May 20, 2024.

4. Arain M, Haque M, Johal L, et al. Maturation of the adolescent brain. *Neuropsychiatr Dis Treat.* 2013;9: 449–461. https://doi.org/10.2147/NDT.S39776
5. Zeoli AM, Goldstick J, Mauri A, et al. The association of firearm laws with firearm outcomes among children and adolescents: a scoping review. *J Behav Med.* 2019;42(4):741–762. https://doi.org/10.1007/s10865-019-00063-y
6. Webster DW, Vernick JS, Zeoli AM, Manganello JA. Association between youth-focused firearm laws and youth suicides. *JAMA.* 2004;292(5):594–601. https://doi.org/10.1001/jama.292.5.594
7. Marvell TB. The impact of banning juvenile gun possession. *J Law Econ.* 2001;44(suppl 2): 691–713. https://doi.org/10.1086/323314
8. Rosengart M, Cummings P, Nathens A, Heagerty P, Maier R, Rivara F. An evaluation of state firearm regulations and homicide and suicide death rates. *Inj Prev.* 2005;11(2):77–83. https://doi.org/10.1136/ip.2004.007062
9. Gius M. The impact of minimum age and child access prevention laws on firearm-related youth suicides and unintentional deaths. *Soc Sci J.* 2015; 52(2):168–175. https://doi.org/10.1016/j.soscij.2015.01.003
10. Kappelman J, Fording RC. The effect of state gun laws on youth suicide by firearm: 1981–2017. *Suicide Life Threat Behav.* 2021;51(2):368–377. https://doi.org/10.1111/sltb.12713
11. Raifman J, Larson E, Barry CL, et al. State handgun purchase age minimums in the US and adolescent suicide rates: regression discontinuity and difference-in-differences analyses. *BMJ.* 2020; 370:m2436. https://doi.org/10.1136/bmj.m2436
12. Rowhani-Rahbar A, Haviland MJ, Ellyson AM. Firearm policy and youth suicide—in pursuit of mechanistic explanations. *JAMA Netw Open.* 2020; 3(11):e2024920. https://doi.org/10.1001/jamanetworkopen.2020.24920
13. Siegel M. *State Firearms Laws in Boston, MA.* Princeton, NJ: Robert Wood Johnson Foundation; 2020.
14. Azrael D, Cook PJ, Miller M. State and local prevalence of firearms ownership: Measurement, structure, and trends. *J Quant Criminol.* 2004;20(1):43–62. https://doi.org/10.1023/B:JOQC.0000016699.11995.c7
15. Auersperg F, Vlasak T, Ponocny I, Barth A. Long-term effects of parental divorce on mental health—a meta-analysis. *J Psychiatr Res.* 2019;119:107–115. https://doi.org/10.1016/j.jpsychires.2019.09.011
16. Siegel M, Ross CS, King C. The relationship between gun ownership and firearm homicide rates in the United States, 1981–2010. *Am J Public Health.* 2013;103(11):2098–2105. https://doi.org/10.2105/AJPH.2013.301409
17. Liang K-Y, Zeger SL. Longitudinal data analysis using linear generalized models. *Biometrika.* 1986; 73(1):13–22. https://doi.org/10.1093/biomet/73.1.13
18. Allison PD, Waterman RP. Fixed-effects negative binomial regression models. *Sociol Methodol.* 2002; 32(1):247–265. https://doi.org/10.1111/1467-9531.00117
19. Schell TL, Peterson S, Vegetabile BG, Scherling A, Smart R, Morral AR. *State-Level Estimates of Household Firearm Ownership.* Santa Monica, CA: RAND; 2020. https://doi.org/10.7249/TL354
20. Smart R, Schell TL, Cefalu M, Morral AR. Impact on nonfirearm deaths of firearm laws affecting firearm deaths: a systematic review and meta-analysis. *Am J Public Health.* 2020;110(10):1–9. https://doi.org/10.2105/AJPH.2020.305808
21. Hanlon TJ, Barber C, Azrael D, Miller M. Type of firearm used in suicides: findings from 13 states in the National Violent Death Reporting System, 2005–2015. *J Adolesc Health.* 2019;65(3):366–370. https://doi.org/10.1016/j.jadohealth.2019.03.015
22. Nestadt PS, MacKrell K, McCourt AD, Fowler DR, Crifasi CK. Prevalence of long gun use in Maryland firearm suicides. *Inj Epidemiol.* 2020;7(4):1–10. https://doi.org/10.1186/s40621-019-0230-y
23. Choi NG, DiNitto DM, Marti CN. Youth firearm suicide: precipitating/risk factors and gun access. *Child Youth Serv Rev.* 2017;83:9–16. https://doi.org/10.1016/j.childyouth.2017.10.022
24. Crifasi CK, Meyers JS, Vernick JS, Webster DW. Effects of changes in permit-to-purchase handgun laws in Connecticut and Missouri on suicide rates. *Prev Med.* 2015;79:43–49. https://doi.org/10.1016/j.ypmed.2015.07.013
25. McCourt AD, Crifasi CK, Stuart EA, et al. Purchaser licensing, point-of-sale background check laws, and firearm homicide and suicide in 4 US states, 1985–2017. *Am J Public Health.* 2020;110(10): 1546–1552. https://doi.org/10.2105/AJPH.2020.305822
26. Crifasi CK, Merrill-Francis M, McCourt A, Vernick JS, Wintemute GJ, Webster DW. Association between firearm laws and homicide in urban counties. *J Urban Health.* 2018;95(3):383–390. https://doi.org/10.1007/s11524-018-0273-3
27. Li M, Small D, Ye T, Lin Y, Webster D. Examining a hypothesized causal chain for the effects of the 2007 repeal of the permit-to-purchase licensing law in Missouri: homicide guns recovered in state within a year of purchase. *J Urban Health.* 2023;100(3):425–430. https://doi.org/10.1007/s11524-023-00739-6
28. Kagawa RM, Castillo-Carniglia A, Vernick JS, et al. Repeal of comprehensive background check policies and firearm homicide and suicide. *Epidemiology.* 2018;29(4):494–502. https://doi.org/10.1097/EDE.0000000000000838
29. Siegel M, Xuan Z, Ross CS, et al. Easiness of legal access to concealed firearm permits and homicide rates in the United States. *Am J Public Health.* 2017;107(12):1923–1929. https://doi.org/10.2105/AJPH.2017.304057
30. Deisenhammer EA, Ing C-M, Strauss R, Kemmler G, Hinterhuber H, Weiss EM. The duration of the suicidal process: how much time is left for intervention between consideration and accomplishment of a suicide attempt? *J Clin Psychiatry.* 2009; 70(1):19–24. https://doi.org/10.4088/JCP.07m03904
31. Rimkeviciene J, O'Gorman J, De Leo D. Impulsive suicide attempts: a systematic literature review of definitions, characteristics, and risk factors. *J Affect Disord.* 2015;171:93–104. https://doi.org/10.1016/j.jad.2014.08.044
32. Barry CL, Stone EM, Crifasi CK, Vernick JS, Webster DW, McGinty EE. Trends in public opinion on US gun laws: majorities of gun owners and non-gun owners support a range of measures. *Health Aff (Millwood).* 2019;38(10):1727–1734. https://doi.org/10.1377/hlthaff.2019.00576

Alcohol Advertising Exposure and Drinking Habits Among Chinese Adolescents in 2021: A National Survey

Ning Ji, PhD, Qingqing Xu, MPH, Xinying Zeng, MPH, Sally Casswell, PhD, Yamin Bai, MPH, and Shiwei Liu, PhD

See also Fang, p. 763.

Objectives. To assess the exposure of Chinese adolescents to proalcohol advertising and explore its association with alcohol consumption.

Methods. A nationally and regionally representative school-based survey was conducted in mainland China in 2021 among students in grades 7 through 12, aged 13 to 18 years. We assessed adolescent exposure to proalcohol advertising and its association with alcohol consumption.

Results. A total of 57 336 students participated in the survey, and the exposure percentage of proalcohol advertising was 66.8%, with no difference between boys and girls or between urban and rural areas. The top 3 exposure channels were television (51.8%), the Internet (43.6%), and outdoor billboards (42.0%). The exposure was higher among students who had consumed alcohol in the past 30 days (80.1% vs 65.1%; adjusted odds ratio [AOR] = 1.29) and in the past 12 months (77.3% vs 61.7%; AOR = 1.30). However, no significant correlation was observed between advertising exposure and drunkenness.

Conclusions. Approximately two thirds of Chinese adolescents have been exposed to proalcohol advertising in the past 30 days, with television, the Internet, and outdoor billboards being the most prevalent channels. Exposure to proalcohol advertising exhibits a positive correlation with drinking.
(*Am J Public Health*. 2024;114(8):814–823. https://doi.org/10.2105/AJPH.2024.307680)

AJPH August 2024, Vol. 114, No. 8

Adolescent drinking is associated with a variety of harmful behaviors and injuries, such as unplanned sex, violence, acute liver disease, and traffic injuries.[1,2] In addition, youth drinking is associated with lifestyle drinking patterns in adulthood and lifelong health problems.[3,4] Alcohol advertising activities increase alcohol consumption and usage,[5] especially engaging the youth familiar with alcohol.[6] Studies have shown a causal relationship between exposure to alcohol advertising and youth initiation and continuation of alcohol consumption.[7,8]

Alcohol has become a serious public health problem in China and directly affects many of the health-related targets of the Sustainable Development Goals (SDGs)[9] and Healthy China 2030.[10] A nationwide survey conducted in 2018 showed that the prevalence of alcohol consumption in the past 12 months among Chinese adults was 39.8% (60.3% for men, 19.1% for women).[11] Alcohol was estimated to be the eighth (fifth among men) leading risk factor in China in terms of disability-adjusted life years (DALYs). It accounted for 4.83% of all deaths and 4.52% of all DALYs in China, which is higher than the global average. Furthermore, about 40% of adolescent deaths in China were attributed to alcohol use.[12]

Marketing of alcohol has grown rapidly since China's reform and opening up in the 1980s.[13] The management of alcohol advertising in China is now mainly based on 2 policies—namely, the Advertising Law of the People's Republic of China[14] (thereafter "Advertising Law") and the Regulation on Broadcasting of Radio and Television Advertisements[15] (thereafter "Broadcasting Regulation"). These 2 policies partially regulate alcohol advertising by stipulating the content, time, and frequency of advertising, and protection of minors. However, there are no provisions regarding outdoor alcohol advertising, and there are currently no regulations for new forms of digital alcohol marketing, including Internet marketing. The Internet and electronic devices such as smartphones are ubiquitous in China. China has 191 billion adolescent Internet users, with a penetration rate of 96.8%.[16] In short, China's current polices on alcohol advertising are incomplete and lag behind new advertising techniques. Moreover, these policies in place were poorly enforced. Scientific information on adolescent exposure to alcohol advertising should help increase our understanding and, thus, help to address the challenge.

There are no data on adolescent exposure to alcohol advertising in mainland China to date. We aimed to provide nationally representative estimates of alcohol advertising exposure and examine its association with alcohol consumption.

METHODS

The target population of this study was all middle- (grades 7–9, ages 13–15 years) and high-school students (grades 10–12, ages 16–18 years) in mainland China. The survey was conducted in 2021 by adopting a multistage stratified cluster probability sampling method. First, 7 provinces from 7 geographic regions in mainland China were selected. Second, the probability proportionate to size sampling was performed; 5 districts and 5 counties were selected in each province. Third, within each selected district or county, 3 middle schools, 2 academic high schools, and 1 vocational high school were randomly selected. Fourth, 1 class was randomly selected from each grade in each school. All students in the selected class completed a self-report survey.

Measures

Respondents were asked if they had seen any advertisements or signs promoting alcohol products in various venues and media during the past 30 days. Venues and media included television, outdoor billboards, newspapers or magazines, the Internet, and sports events, community events, concerts, or fairs (thereafter "events"). Responses were coded as "1 = No access to the venue/media in the previous 30 days"; "2 = never"; "3 = sometimes"; or "4 = often." Responses coded 3 and 4 were considered exposed. The exposure to alcohol advertising was measured based on the exposure of the 5 types of exposure. Exposure to any of the 5 types was classified as exposed, while no exposure in all 5 types was categorized as unexposed. Exposure to drinking imagery was measured by the question "During the past 30 days, have you seen an actor/actress drinking alcohol on television, film, recording or video?" Responses were "1 = never"; "2 = sometimes"; "3 = often"; and "4 = always." Responses coded from 2 to 4 were considered exposed.

Both alcohol consumption and drunken state were measured. Alcohol consumption was measured using the question "Have you had at least one drink in the past 12 months? (One drink is equivalent to half a bottle/can of beer, a small cup of white wine, a glass of wine, or a glass of rice wine.)" Responses were "1 = No"; "2 = Yes, before the previous 30 days"; and "3 = Yes, in the previous 30 days." Responses coded 2 were deemed to indicate drinking in the past 30 days, while responses coded 1 and 3 suggested no drinking in this period. In addition, responses coded 2 and 3 were interpreted as indicating drinking in the past 12 months. The drunken state was measured using the question "Have you ever been drunk in the past 12 months? (Drunkenness: A person experiences symptoms such as confusion, slurred speech, vomiting, coma and so on caused by excessive drinking)." Responses were "1 = No"; "2 = Yes, before the previous 30 days"; "3 = Yes, in the previous 30 days"; and "4=Haven't had a drink in the previous 12 months." Responses coded 2 and 3 were considered to indicate having experienced drunkenness within the past 12 months, while those coded 1 and 4 were deemed to indicate no drunkenness.

Statistical Analysis

Accounting for complex sampling, we applied a weighted scheme to all estimations. We determined the total weight of each respondent by 3 weights: the base weight, the nonresponse adjustment weight, and the poststratification adjustment weight. We calculated the base weight by multiplying the primary sampling unit weight (reciprocal of sampling probability by population), the school weight (reciprocal of sampling probability by the number of students), and the class weight (total number of classes for this grade). We obtained the nonresponse adjustment weight by multiplying the reciprocals of the response rates of primary sampling unit, school, class, and student. We computed the poststratification adjustment weight based on the composition of urban–rural, school type, gender, and grade. Based on the final weight, we calculated point percentage and 95% confidence intervals (CIs) for each proportion.[17]

We analyzed the general information of the participants and their exposure to proalcohol advertising. We stratified all estimates by gender, urban or rural residence, grade, school type, and geographic region. We performed the Rao-Scott χ^2 test to compare the differences between groups. We used multilevel logistic regression to explore the relationship between proalcohol advertising exposure and alcohol consumption. Level 2 pertained to schools, while level 1 referred to individual students. We calculated both crude odds ratio (OR) and adjusted odds ratio (AOR). The criterion for statistical difference was a 2-tailed *P* value of < .05. We used SAS version 9.4 (SAS Institute Inc, Cary, NC) SURVEYFREQ and SURVEYLOGISTIC procedures for all statistical computations.

RESULTS

A total of 57 336 students of grades 7 through 12 aged 13 to 18 years participated in the survey (response rate 96.0%). The respondents were from 379 schools in 7 provinces: 7956 in Beijing, 8405 in Guangdong, 5838 in Heilongjiang, 10 440 in Henan, 8942 in Jiangxi, 9596 in Sichuan, and 6159 in Ningxia. Among them, 29 694 were middle-school students, 20 586 were academic high-school students, and 7056 were vocational high-school students. The distribution was similar across grades. Of all students, 51.7% were boys and 59.4% were from urban areas. (Appendix Table A, available as a supplement to the online version of this article at https://ajph.org).

Exposure to Alcohol Advertising

Table 1 presents the exposure to proalcohol advertising among adolescents and ORs of different groups. The prevalence of exposure to proalcohol advertising among students in grades 7 through 12 was 66.8%, with no difference between boys and girls or between urban and rural areas. Exposure prevalence differed among grades, increasing from 55.4% of grade 7 to 73.7% of grade 12. Exposure was lower in middle-school students (62.1%) compared with high-school students (73.0%), with no significant difference between academic and vocational high-school students.

We observed geographic disparities, with relatively high exposure percentages in Southwest China (71.2%) and North China (70.1%), while Northeast China exhibited the lowest level of exposure at 60.8%. The region with the highest advertising exposure for middle-school students was identified in North China at 67.2%, whereas the region with the highest exposure for high-school students was situated in Southwest China at 78.5%. By contrast, Northeast China demonstrated the lowest levels of advertising exposure for both middle-school students (54.7%) and high-school students (67.3%). The geographic distribution showed a similar pattern among academic and vocational high-school students (Table 1, Figure 1, Appendix Table B, and Appendix Figure A).

Types of Alcohol Advertising Exposure

The highest exposure to alcohol advertising was on television (51.8%). This was followed by the Internet (43.6%) and outdoor billboards (42.0%). Exposure was relatively lower in events (22.3%) and newspapers or magazines (20.8%). Among students who had accessed those advertising approaches, television was the most common type (69.1%), followed by billboard (62.5%). Girls were more likely than boys to be exposed through television, billboard, and the Internet, while boys were more likely than girls to be exposed through events. No statistically significant difference was found between urban and rural students across all 5 advertising channels. Additionally, exposure percentages were higher for older students across all channels (Appendix Table C).

The geographic distribution of proalcohol advertising exposure varied across different advertising channels. Among all students, with the exception of the Internet, Southwest China exhibits the highest exposure across the 4 types of channels. The region with the greatest exposure to online advertising is North China. Among those exposed to these advertising channels, Southwest China consistently had the highest exposure in each venue or media. On the other hand, Northeast China or East China had the lowest exposure in various venues or media, both among all students and those exposed to these advertising channels. This geographic distribution pattern of alcohol advertising exposure through different channels was similar among middle- and high-school students, as well as among academic and vocational high-school students (Appendix Table C).

Exposure to Drinking Imagery

Among middle- and high-school students overall, 66.2% reported noticing drinking imagery in the past 30 days. The percentage rose to 81.1% among individuals who had been exposed to television, film, recording, or video. The prevalence of imagery exposure was higher among high-school students (70.7%) compared with middle-school

TABLE 1— Exposure to Alcohol Advertising Among Middle- and High-School Students: China, 2021

	Overall (n = 57 336)			Middle-School Students (n = 29 694)			High-School Students (n = 27 642)		
	Exposed No.	Weighted % (95% CI)	OR (95%CI)	Exposed No.	Weighted % (95% CI)	OR (95%CI)	Exposed No.	Weighted % (95% CI)	OR (95%CI)
Total	38 505	66.8 (65.0, 68.5)		18 402	62.1 (60.2, 64.0)		20 103	73.0 (71.4, 74.6)	
Sex									
Boys	19 738	66.3 (64.8, 67.8)	1 (Ref)	9 520	62.0 (60.1, 63.9)	1 (Ref)	10 218	72.2 (70.8, 73.7)	1 (Ref)
Girls	18 767	67.3 (65.0, 69.6)	1.0 (1.0, 1.1)	8 882	62.1 (60.1, 64.2)	1.0 (1.0, 1.1)	9 885	73.8 (71.0, 76.6)	1.1 (0.9, 1.3)
Residence									
Urban	22 875	67.2 (65.6, 68.8)	1 (Ref)	10 928	63.2 (61.1, 65.3)	1 (Ref)	11 947	72.4 (70.6, 74.2)	1 (Ref)
Rural	15 630	66.5 (63.9, 69.2)	1.0 (0.8, 1.1)	7 474	61.4 (58.7, 64.1)	0.9 (0.8, 1.1)	8 156	73.3 (71.1, 75.6)	1.0 (0.9, 1.2)
Grade									
7	5 623	55.4 (53.5, 57.4)	1 (Ref)	5 623	55.4 (53.5, 57.4)	1 (Ref)			
8	6 299	64.2 (61.3, 67.1)	1.4 (1.2, 1.7)	6 299	64.2 (61.3, 67.1)	1.4 (1.2, 1.7)			
9	6 480	66.9 (64.2, 69.7)	1.6 (1.5, 1.8)	6 480	66.9 (64.2, 69.7)	1.6 (1.5, 1.8)			
10	6 713	71.7 (68.8, 74.6)	2.0 (1.7, 2.4)				6 713	71.7 (68.8, 74.6)	1 (Ref)
11	6 948	73.8 (71.5, 76.1)	2.3 (2.0, 2.6)				6 948	73.8 (71.5, 76.1)	0.9 (0.7, 1.1)
12	6 442	73.7 (70.7, 76.7)	2.3 (2.0, 2.6)				6 442	73.7 (70.7, 76.7)	1.0 (0.9, 1.1)
Region									
Northeast	3 531	60.8 (57.5, 64.0)	1 (Ref)	1 698	54.7 (49.2, 60.1)	1 (Ref)	1 833	67.3 (64.3, 70.3)	1 (Ref)
East	5 456	63.0 (58.6, 67.3)	1.1 (0.9, 1.4)	2 449	57.6 (53.8, 61.4)	1.1 (0.9, 1.5)	3 007	69.9 (66.5, 73.4)	1.1 (0.9, 1.4)
North	5 526	70.1 (68.1, 72.0)	1.5 (1.3, 1.8)	2 653	67.2 (64.0, 70.5)	1.7 (1.3, 2.2)	2 873	74.4 (72.5, 76.3)	1.4 (1.2, 1.7)
Central	7 162	68.0 (63.7, 72.4)	1.4 (1.1, 1.7)	3 517	64.1 (60.2, 68.1)	1.5 (1.1, 2.0)	3 645	73.6 (68.8, 78.5)	1.4 (1.0, 1.8)
South	5 817	67.7 (63.9, 71.5)	1.4 (1.1, 1.7)	2 738	64.1 (60.1, 68.1)	1.5 (1.1, 2.0)	3 079	72.9 (67.6, 78.3)	1.3 (1.0, 1.8)
Northwest	4 142	66.4 (62.4, 70.3)	1.3 (1.0, 1.6)	1 909	61.2 (57.1, 65.4)	1.3 (1.0, 1.7)	2 233	73.0 (68.7, 77.4)	1.3 (1.0, 1.7)
Southwest	6 871	71.2 (68.3, 74.0)	1.6 (1.3, 1.9)	3 438	65.0 (60.6, 69.4)	1.5 (1.2, 2.1)	3 433	78.5 (76.5, 80.5)	1.8 (1.5, 2.1)
Drink in the past 30 d									
No	33 448	65.1 (63.3, 66.9)	1 (Ref)	16 589	60.5 (58.7, 62.3)	1 (Ref)	16 859	71.5 (69.7, 73.3)	1 (Ref)
Yes	5 040	80.1 (78.9, 81.3)	2.2 (1.9, 2.4)	1 801	77.8 (75.9, 79.7)	2.3 (2.1, 2.5)	3 239	82.0 (79.6, 84.5)	1.8 (1.5, 2.2)
Drink in the past 12 mo									
No	24 360	61.7 (59.9, 63.4)	1 (Ref)	12 896	57.5 (55.8, 59.3)	1 (Ref)	11 464	68.5 (66.6, 70.3)	1 (Ref)
Yes	14 128	77.3 (76.1, 78.5)	2.1 (2.0, 2.3)	5 494	74.6 (72.9, 76.4)	2.2 (2.0, 2.4)	8 634	79.5 (77.8, 81.2)	1.8 (1.6, 2.0)
Drunk in the past 12 mo									
No	35 048	66.1 (64.4, 67.8)	1 (Ref)	17 039	61.5 (59.6, 63.3)	1 (Ref)	18 009	72.5 (70.9, 74.0)	1 (Ref)
Yes	2 456	77.8 (76.2, 79.5)	1.8 (1.7, 2.0)	846	74.4 (72.1, 76.7)	1.8 (1.6, 2.1)	1 610	80.1 (77.7, 82.6)	1.5 (1.3, 1.8)

Note. CI = confidence interval; OR = odds ratio.

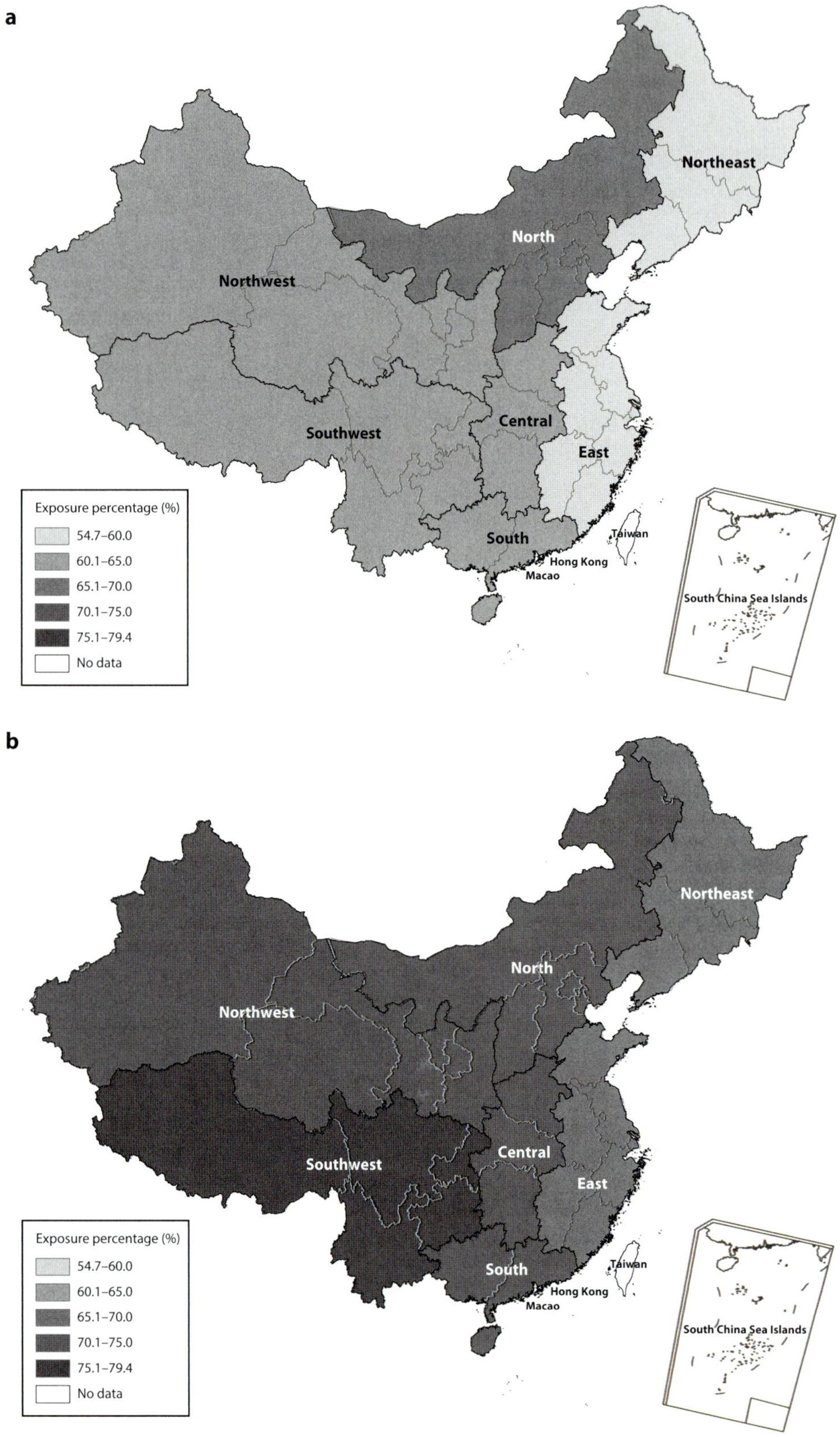

FIGURE 1— Geographical Disparities in Alcohol Advertising Exposure Among (a) Middle- and (b) High-School Students: China, 2021

students (62.9%). In middle-school students, the exposure to drinking imagery increased progressively with grade level, whereas there was no statistically significant variation across different grades in high-school students. Vocational high-school students had higher exposure in rural areas compared with urban areas. The highest exposure to drinking imagery was found in Central China at 68.0%, while the lowest exposure was found in Northeast China at 57.4%. Compared with Northeast China, exposure percentages in other geographical regions were significantly higher, but there were no statistical differences within them (Appendix Table D).

Alcohol Advertising and Adolescent Drinking

According to Table 1, the percentage of proalcohol advertising exposure was higher among students who had consumed alcohol in the past 30 days (80.1% vs 65.1%) and in the past 12 months (77.3% vs 61.7%), compared with nondrinkers during those respective periods. The association between exposure to proalcohol advertising and alcohol consumption among middle- and high-school students exhibited a consistent pattern. After controlling for 9 adjusting variables—gender, urban–rural residence, school type, pocket money, cigarette use status, parent alcohol use status, friend alcohol use status, and exposure to antialcohol information—significant correlations remained between alcohol advertising exposure and alcohol consumption within the past 30 days (AOR = 1.29) as well as in the previous 12 months (AOR = 1.30). There was no statistically significant association between exposure to alcohol advertising and drunkenness (Table 2).

DISCUSSION

This survey is the first nationally representative survey on alcohol advertising exposure of adolescents in China. Our findings revealed that, in 2021, the

TABLE 2— Relationship Between Alcohol Advertising Exposure and Alcohol Consumption Among Middle- and High-School Students: China, 2021

Independent Value	Drink in the Past 30 Days, AOR (95% CI)	Drink in the Past 12 Months, AOR (95% CI)	Drunk in the Past 12 Months, AOR (95% CI)
Exposed to alcohol advertising: yes (Ref = no)	1.29 (1.02, 1.62)	1.30 (1.08, 1.57)	1.26 (0.99, 1.61)
Sex: girls (Ref = boys)	0.57 (0.42, 0.79)	0.82 (0.66, 1.03)	0.58 (0.31, 1.11)
Residence: rural (Ref = urban)	1.48 (1.19, 1.83)	1.34 (1.14, 1.57)	1.78 (1.23, 2.56)
School			
Academic high school (Ref = middle school)	0.96 (0.75, 1.23)	1.09 (0.92, 1.29)	1.28 (0.83, 1.98)
Vocational high school	0.96 (0.74, 1.24)	0.94 (0.79, 1.11)	1.97 (1.28, 3.03)
Pocket money: RMB, ¥ (Ref = 0)			
≤ 10	1.41 (0.58, 3.40)	1.07 (0.93, 1.24)	3.23 (0.88, 11.8)
11–30	1.19 (0.76, 1.88)	1.06 (0.80, 1.39)	1.59 (1.00, 2.54)
31–50	1.84 (1.04, 3.26)	1.68 (1.50, 1.89)	3.80 (1.95, 7.42)
> 50	2.92 (1.35, 6.31)	1.86 (1.52, 2.26)	1.96 (1.09, 3.52)
Cigarette use status: yes (Ref = no)	3.19 (2.45, 4.15)	5.68 (3.65, 8.85)	4.13 (2.96, 5.77)
E-cigarette use status: yes (Ref = no)	1.56 (1.05, 2.31)	1.77 (1.08, 2.90)	3.04 (2.18, 4.25)
Parent alcohol use			
Father or mother (Ref = neither father nor mother)	1.88 (1.28, 2.75)	1.68 (1.25, 2.25)	1.24 (0.85, 1.81)
Both father and mother	2.27 (1.05, 4.89)	1.70 (1.20, 2.40)	1.29 (0.62, 2.69)
Friend alcohol use			
Some (Ref = none)	8.48 (3.11, 23.11)	6.45 (4.04, 10.32)	2.82 (2.01, 3.94)
Almost all or all	17.57 (6.69, 46.16)	21.66 (9.36, 50.16)	7.61 (4.62, 12.56)
Heard or seen information that drinking is harmful to health: yes (Ref = no)	0.99 (0.67, 1.46)	0.86 (0.79, 0.93)	0.97 (0.83, 1.15)

Note. AOR = adjusted odds ratio; CI = confidence interval; RMB = renminbi. The multilevel logistic regression model was used, with level 2 representing schools and level 1 denoting individual students. Adjusted variables included sex, residence and school, pocket money, cigarette use status, parent alcohol use status, friend alcohol use status, and heard or seen information that drinking is harmful to health.

exposure percentage to proalcohol advertising in the past 30 days among Chinese adolescents aged 13 to 18 years was 66.8%. This indicates that the exposure to proalcohol advertising among Chinese adolescents is prevalent. Similar to the pattern of exposure to protobacco advertising among Chinese adolescents[18] and proalcohol advertising in Australia,[19] the primary means of exposure to proalcohol advertising were through television, followed by outdoor billboards and the Internet. A study conducted in the United States revealed that girls are exposed to a significantly higher degree of alcohol advertising compared with boys.[20] However, when examining Chinese adolescents, we found no statistically significant disparity in the proportion of boys and girls exposed to alcohol advertisements. Nevertheless, it is worth noting that the exposure of girls to proalcohol advertising through television, billboards, and the Internet is considerably higher than that of boys.

The primary basis for regulation of alcohol advertising in China, namely the Advertising Law, stipulates that alcohol advertisements shall not contain the following information: inducing or encouraging drinking or promoting excessive drinking; drinking imagery; performing activities such as driving a car, boat, airplane, etc.; and expressing or implying a message that drinking eliminates tension and anxiety, increases physical strength, and so on. In addition, the Broadcasting Management Measures specify the quantity of alcohol advertising. Our findings revealed that television is the primary medium for proalcohol advertising exposure across gender, residence, region, grade, and school type. About 1 in 2 students reported exposure to proalcohol product advertisements on television within the past 30 days, and among those who watched television, the percentage was about 70%. The high exposure of alcohol advertising on television is likely attributable to the widespread availability of television in China, with 97.0% of Chinese households owning a television. This also indicates that the current policies in place, which aim to prevent the advertising of alcohol products to minors, are not effective.

In China, virtually every adolescent is an Internet user. Our findings indicate that exposure to alcohol advertising was second highest through the Internet (43.6%). Among Internet users, the proportion reached 54.1%. Currently, China regulates Internet advertising in accordance with the Interim Administrative Measures on Internet Advertising.[21] However, these measures do not include any provisions specifically addressing alcohol advertising, unlike tobacco advertising, which is prohibited. Our findings also show that adolescents are exposed to online alcohol advertising to a greater extent than tobacco advertising.[22] In 2020, Internet advertising comprised around 60% of the total size of China's advertising market.[23] Considering the extensive Internet accessibility and the rapid expansion of Internet advertising in China, it would be beneficial to incorporate a comprehensive ban on alcohol advertising into the Interim Administrative Measures on Internet Advertising, mirroring the approach taken for tobacco advertising online.

In China, outdoor billboards (42.0%) ranked as the third most prevalent medium for exposure to alcohol advertising. Among students who had accessed the Internet or billboards, the proportion of exposure to alcohol advertising from outdoor billboards (62.5%) was higher than that from the Internet (54.1%). Previously, outdoor advertising in China was governed by the Regulations on the Registration and Administration of Outdoor Advertising,[24] but the regulation was repealed in 2016. Since then, outdoor advertising in China has been regulated under the Advertising Law. However, the law does not contain specific provisions regarding outdoor advertising, let alone on outdoor alcohol advertising. As a conventional advertising channel, outdoor advertising is also growing with the rapid development of China's economy. Although the overall growth rate has slowed down because of the rise of the Internet advertising, the integration of digital outdoor advertising shows a new trend. Therefore, outdoor alcohol advertising must also be given due attention.

Approximately 20% of adolescents reported exposure to proalcohol advertising via newspapers or magazines or events, which is significantly lower than through television, the Internet, or outdoor billboards. The exposure to proalcohol advertising among Chinese adolescents mirrors the pattern observed in tobacco advertising,[18] with each channel having a substantial advertising exposure percentage. Notably, the platform with the lowest exposure to proalcohol advertising, namely newspapers or magazines (20.8%), exhibits a comparable exposure percentage to the platform with the highest exposure to protobacco advertising, which is television (21.3%), among Chinese adolescents.

Studies have shown that portrayal of alcohol consumption in media can affect the attitudes and norms of adolescents,[25] initiate drinking among youths,[26] and guide imitative drinking behavior.[27] Therefore, the Advertising

Law stipulates that alcohol advertisements should not contain scenes of drinking. However, this survey found that a significant majority of students (81.1%) had been exposed to portrayals of drinking among those who had watched television, videos, or movies in the past 30 days. Our findings are consistent with several studies, including a content analysis of TikTok's top 100 popular videos, which revealed that 72% of these videos featured liquor,[28] indicating that the portrayal of drinking scenes is highly prevalent in today's media. These results emphasize the imperative for stricter enforcement and improvement of pertinent laws.

One notable finding of this study was the geographical disparity in exposure to alcohol advertising. The region with the lowest prevalence of exposure to alcohol advertising, alcohol advertisements on television and billboards, and alcohol-related imagery is primarily situated in Northeast China, which has the lowest socioeconomic status. Conversely, the highest proportion of these indicators is primarily observed in Southwest China, which has a middle socioeconomic status. The findings suggest that variations in the geographical distribution of alcohol advertising exposure may be influenced by factors beyond economic levels alone. The lower exposure observed in the northeast region, besides being influenced by local economic conditions, could also be attributed to the colder climate resulting in reduced outdoor activities and subsequently less exposure to outdoor alcohol advertisements. Conversely, the high exposure observed in Southwest China may be attributed to the more slow-paced and leisurely lifestyle in this locality.

The positive association between proalcohol advertising and adolescent alcohol consumption has been extensively investigated. A study conducted on 909 Chilean adolescents revealed that recent exposure to alcohol advertising increased the likelihood of alcohol consumption by 41% and posed an elevated risk of problematic drinking by up to 85%.[29] According to a cross-sectional study involving 3806 school children in Cambodia, daily or near-daily exposure to alcohol advertising was linked with current drinking (OR = 1.6) and drunkenness (OR = 2.3).[30] Our study provides further evidence for these findings, as it reveals that, after controlling for 9 covariates, students who had consumed alcohol within the past 30 days (AOR = 1.29) and those who drank within the past 12 months (AOR = 1.30) were significantly more likely to be exposed to advertisements promoting alcohol compared with their counterparts who did not consume alcohol in the past year. Interestingly, no statistically significant association was observed between exposure to alcohol advertisements and drunkenness. This may be attributed to the influence of multiple factors on drunkenness, such as temperamental, socioeconomic, and family factors.[31]

Strengths and Limitations

This study had several strengths. It used a large-scale survey utilizing complex sampling and weighted estimation, ensuring national, regional, and provincial representativeness. The study estimated the exposure to proalcohol advertising among Chinese adolescents and examined its association with alcohol consumption. It serves as a baseline for future research on the overexposure of youths to alcohol advertising.

This study was subject to 2 main limitations. First, the information was gathered using self-reported paper questionnaires, which may introduce recall bias. However, the large sample size of this study helped to mitigate the impact of this bias in practice. Second, given that this was a cross-sectional study, although a positive correlation was observed between exposure to alcohol advertising and adolescent drinking, it was unable to establish a causal relationship between alcohol exposure and increased drinking or imply that adolescents who consume alcohol were more attentive to alcohol advertisements. Nonetheless, the large sample size and adjustment with 9 variables in this study ensured the stability of the observed associations.

Public Health Implications

This study highlights the concerning issue of proalcohol advertising exposure among Chinese adolescents. The multichannel exposure pattern, including television, the Internet, and outdoor billboards, observed among Chinese adolescents indicates that restrictions solely targeting specific media types are insufficient. When only certain categories of proalcohol advertising are restricted, it may lead to an expansion of alternative media types used for advertising purposes.

Bans or comprehensive restrictions on alcohol advertising have been implemented in various countries. For example, Finland introduced policies aimed at reducing young people's exposure to alcohol advertising by imposing limitations on timing and placement. These measures included banning alcohol advertisements on television between 7:00 and 19:00 and in cinemas, as well as prohibiting alcohol advertising on social media.[32] Subsequently, other countries such as Brunei and Lithuania also adopted similar policies, leading to a growing number of nations with total or near-total bans on alcohol advertising.[33] The practices implemented by these countries, in conjunction with the recommendations from the World Health Organization,[34] serve as valuable reference experiences for enhancing our policies.

Considering the challenges in limiting alcohol advertisements to only reach young adults and avoid reaching underage individuals, the most optimal strategy for China would be to implement a comprehensive ban on alcohol advertising. Currently, the responsibility for monitoring and enforcing the existing regulations on advertising in China primarily lies with the administrative department for industry and commerce. This is coordinated with various other administrative departments, including health, food and drug, cultural tourism, industrialization and information technology, and natural resources, as well as the National Radio and Television Administration. In addition to the multi-department management of advertising supervision, the low penalties in the case of violation, the lack of effective detection, and vested interests of some organizations all hinder the effective implementation of the partial regulations to some extent.

To address the aforementioned challenges, targeted measures can be implemented, such as clarifying the enforcement agencies and developing advertising detection technologies. These actions will strengthen the implementation of strategies and subsequently reduce the exposure of young people to alcohol advertising. AJPH

ABOUT THE AUTHORS

Ning Ji and Yamin Bai are with the National Center for Chronic and Noncommunicable Disease Control and Prevention, Chinese Center for Disease Control and Prevention, Beijing, China. Qingqing Xu is with the Zaozhuang Center for Disease Control and Prevention, Zaozhuang, Shandong, China. Xinying Zeng and Shiwei Liu are with the Tobacco Control Office, Chinese Center for Disease Control and Prevention. Sally Casswell is with the Social and Health Outcomes Research and Evaluation (SHORE), SHORE and Whariki Research Centre, College of Health, Massey University, Auckland, New Zealand.

CORRESPONDENCE

Correspondence should be sent to Shiwei Liu, PhD, Tobacco Control Office, Chinese Center for Disease Control and Prevention, 27# Nanwei Road, Xicheng District, Beijing 100050, China (e-mail: shiwei_liu@aliyun.com); or Yamin Bai, MPH, National Center for Chronic and Noncommunicable Disease Control and Prevention, Chinese Center for Disease Control and Prevention, 27# Nanwei Road, Xicheng District, Beijing 100050, China (e-mail: baiyamin@ncncd.chinacdc.cn). Reprints can be ordered at https://www.ajph.org by clicking the "Reprints" link.

PUBLICATION INFORMATION

Full Citation: Ji N, Xu Q, Zeng X, Casswell S, Bai Y, Liu S. Alcohol advertising exposure and drinking habits among Chinese adolescents in 2021: a national survey. *Am J Public Health*. 2024;114(8): 814–823.

Acceptance Date: March 29, 2024.

DOI: https://doi.org/10.2105/AJPH.2024.307680

ORCID iD:

Ning Ji https://orcid.org/0000-0001-5405-2584

CONTRIBUTORS

S. Liu and Y. Bai conceptualized the study. X. Zeng conducted the data collection and visualization. S. Liu and S. Casswell supervised data interpretation. N. Ji and Q. Xu analyzed the data and drafted the article. All authors provided critical feedback. N. Ji and Q. Xu are co-first authors and have contributed equally to this work. S. Liu and Y. Bai have contributed equally and share the position of co-corresponding authors.

CONFLICTS OF INTEREST

The authors have no conflicts of interest to report.

HUMAN PARTICIPANT PROTECTION

The institutional review board of Chinese Center for Disease Control and Prevention approved the study (No. 202115), and consent was obtained from school officials and respondents.

REFERENCES

1. Hingson RW, Zha W. Binge drinking above and below twice the adolescent thresholds and health-risk behaviors. *Alcohol Clin Exp Res*. 2018; 42(5):904–913. https://doi.org/10.1111/acer.13627
2. Prasartpornsirichoke J, Kalayasiri R, Vichitkunakorn P, et al. Association of supply sources of alcohol and alcohol-related harms in adolescent drinkers: the baseline characteristics of a high school cohort across Thailand. *BMC Public Health*. 2022;22(1):2277. https://doi.org/10.1186/s12889-022-14767-5
3. Soundararajan S, Narayanan G, Agrawal A, Prabhakaran D, Murthy P. Relation between age at first alcohol drink adult life drinking patterns in alcohol-dependent patients. *Indian J Med Res*. 2017;146:606–611.
4. Dawson DA, Goldstein RB, Chou SP, Ruan WJ, Grant BF. Age at first drink and the first incidence of adult-onset *DSM-IV* alcohol use disorders. *Alcohol Clin Exp Res*. 2008;32(12):2149–2160. https://doi.org/10.1111/j.1530-0277.2008.00806.x
5. Niederdeppe J, Avery RJ, Tabor E, Lee NW, Welch B, Skurka C. Estimated televised alcohol advertising exposure in the past year and associations with past 30-day drinking behavior among American adults: results from a secondary analysis of large-scale advertising and survey data. *Addiction*. 2021;116(2):280–289. https://doi.org/10.1111/add.15088
6. Ibitoye M, Kaaya S, Parker R, Likindikoki S, Ngongi L, Sommer M. The influence of alcohol outlet density and advertising on youth drinking in urban Tanzania. *Health Place*. 2019;58:102141. https://doi.org/10.1016/j.healthplace.2019.05.019
7. Weitzman M, Lee L. Similarities between alcohol and tobacco advertising exposure and adolescent use of each of these substances. *J Stud Alcohol Drugs Suppl*. 2020;19(suppl 19):97–105. https://doi.org/10.15288/jsads.2020.s19.97
8. Padon AA, Rimal RN, Siegel M, DeJong W, Naimi TS, JernFigan DH. Alcohol brand use of youth-appealing advertising and consumption by youth and adults. *J Public Health Res*. 2018;7(1):1269. https://doi.org/10.4081/jphr.2018.1269
9. United Nations Department of Economic and Social Affairs. Sustainable Development Goals. 2015. Available at: https://sdgs.un.org/goals. Accessed November 18, 2022.
10. The Communist Party of China Central Committee and the State Council. "Healthy China 2030" Blueprint. 2016. Available at: http://www.gov.cn/xinwen/2016-10/25/content_5124174.htm. Accessed November 22, 2022.
11. Chinese Center for Disease Control and Prevention. *Report on Chronic Disease Risk Factor Surveillance in China, 2018*. Beijing, China: People's Health Publishing House; 2021.
12. GBD 2019 Risk Factors Collaborators. Global burden of 87 risk factors in 204 countries and territories, 1990–2019: a systematic analysis for the Global Burden of Disease Study 2019. *Lancet*. 2020;396(10258):1223–1249. https://doi.org/10.1016/S0140-6736(20)30752-2
13. Liu S, Huang F, Zhu X, et al. China's changing alcohol market and need for an enhanced policy response: a narrative review. *Int J Environ Res Public Health*. 2022;19(10):5866. https://doi.org/10.3390/ijerph19105866
14. The National People's Congress. Advertisement law of the People's Republic of China. 2015. Available at: http://www.npc.gov.cn/npc/cwhhy/12jcwh/2015-04/25/content_1934594.htm. Accessed May 15, 2023.
15. The State Council of the People's Republic of China. Order no. 61 of the national radio and television administration: regulation on

broadcasting of radio and television advertisements. 2009. Available at: http://www.gov.cn/flfg/2009-09/10/content_1414069.htm. Accessed December 15, 2022.

16. China Internet Network Information Center. Report on Internet use among Chinese minors in 2021. 2022. Available at: https://www.cnnic.cn/n4/2022/1201/c116-10690.html. Accessed May 10, 2023.

17. Zhao Y, Di XB, Li SX, et al. Prevalence, frequency, intensity, and location of cigarette use among adolescents in China from 2013–14 to 2019: findings from two repeated cross-sectional studies. *Lancet Reg Health West Pac*; 2022:27:100549. https://doi.org/10.1016/j.lanwpc.2022.100549

18. Xiao L, Yang J, Zhao L, Jiang Y, Chen X. Exposure to tobacco advertisement and promotion programs among Chinese middle school students: a cross-sectional survey [in Chinese]. *Zhonghua Liu Xing Bing Xue Za Zhi.* 2015;36(4):309–313.

19. Bain E, Scully M, Wakefield M, Durkin S, White V. Association between single-channel and cumulative exposure to alcohol advertising and drinking behaviours among Australian adolescents. *Drug Alcohol Rev.* 2023;42(1):59–67. https://doi.org/10.1111/dar.13530

20. Collins RL, Martino SC, Kovalchik SA, Becker KM, Shadel WG, D'Amico EJ. Alcohol advertising exposure among middle school-age youth: an assessment across all media and venues. *J Stud Alcohol Drugs.* 2016;77(3):384–392. https://doi.org/10.15288/jsad.2016.77.384

21. The State Council of the People's Republic of China. Order No. 87 of the State Administration for Industry and Commerce of the People's Republic of China: interim regulation on the administration of Internet advertising. 2016. Available at: http://www.gov.cn/xinwen/2016-07/09/content_5089902.htm. Accessed February 25, 2023.

22. Xi Z, Di XB, Nan Y, et al. Analysis of exposure to tobacco advertisement and promotion among Chinese adults aged 15 years and above, 2010 and 2018 [in Chinese]. *Zhonghua Liu Xing Bing Xue Za Zhi.* 2022;43(6):830–834.

23. Sun X. Trend analysis of the Internet advertising industry operation and development [in Chinese]. *China's National Conditions and Strength.* 2022(1):9–16.

24. The State Council of the People's Republic of China. Order No. 25 of the State Administration for Industry and Commerce of the People's Republic of China: regulations on the administration of outdoor advertisement registration. 2006. Available at: http://www.gov.cn/ziliao/flfg/2006-06/07/content_302493.htm. Accessed February 25, 2023.

25. Merrill JE, López G, Doucette H, et al. Adolescents' perceptions of alcohol portrayals in the media and their impact on cognitions and behaviors. *Psychol Addict Behav.* 2023;37(6):758–770. https://doi.org/10.1037/adb0000907

26. Bigman G, Wilkinson AV, Vandewater EA, et al. Viewing images of alcohol use in PG-13-rated movies and alcohol initiation in Mexican-heritage youth. *J Ethn Subst Abuse.* 2020;19(4):521–536. https://doi.org/10.1080/15332640.2018.1548319

27. Bleakley A, Ellithorpe ME, Hennessy M, Khurana A, Jamieson P, Weitz I. Alcohol, sex, and screens: modeling media influence on adolescent alcohol and sex co-occurrence. *J Sex Res.* 2017;54(8):1026–1037. https://doi.org/10.1080/00224499.2017.1279585

28. Russell AM, Davis RE, Ortega JM, Colditz JB, Primack B, Barry AE. #Alcohol: portrayals of alcohol in top videos on TikTok. *J Stud Alcohol Drugs.* 2021;82(5):615–622. https://doi.org/10.15288/jsad.2021.82.615

29. Sanhueza GE, Delva J, Bares CB, Grogan-Kaylor A. Alcohol consumption among Chilean adolescents: examining individual, peer, parenting and environmental factors. *Int J Alcohol Drug Res.* 2013;2(1):89–97. https://doi.org/10.7895/ijadr.v2i1.71

30. Peltzer K, Pengpid S, Tepirou C. Associations of alcohol use with mental health and alcohol exposure among school-going students in Cambodia. *Nagoya J Med Sci.* 2016;78(4):415–422.

31. Enstad F, Pedersen W, Nilsen W, von Soest T. Predicting early onset of intoxication versus drinking—a population-based prospective study of Norwegian adolescents. *Addict Behav Rep.* 2017;6:1–7. https://doi.org/10.1016/j.abrep.2017.04.002

32. Katainen A, Kauppila E, Svensson J, Lindeman M, Hellman M. Regulating alcohol marketing on social media: outcomes and limitations of marketing restrictions of Finland's 2015 Alcohol Act. *J Stud Alcohol Drugs.* 2020;81(1):39–46. https://doi.org/10.15288/jsad.2020.81.39

33. Herrera Amul GG. Alcohol advertising, promotion, and sponsorship: a review of regulatory policies in the Association of Southeast Asian Nations. *J Stud Alcohol Drugs.* 2020;81(6):697–709. https://doi.org/10.15288/jsad.2020.81.697

34. World Health Organization. The SAFER initiative. 2018. Available at: https://www.who.int/initiatives/SAFER. Accessed December 1, 2022.

"The Hotel of 10,000 Stars": The Impact of Social-Structural Determinants of Health Among Im/migrant Shrimpers in the Gulf of Mexico

Shannon Guillot-Wright, PhD, Lacy Davis, MA, Linh Truong, PA-C, Heide Castañeda, PhD, and Anabel Rodriguez, PhD

Objectives. To identify appropriate interventions to prevent injury, we conducted a qualitative study among commercial shrimp fishermen in the Gulf of Mexico.

Methods. Using qualitative and participatory research methods, including interviews, photovoice, and workplace observations in southeast Texas and the Rio Grande Valley in Texas, we examined the social–structural dimensions that contribute to physical and psychological injury.

Results. We found that multiple layers of vulnerability and danger exist among shrimpers with interacting themes: (1) recognizing risk, (2) precarious employment, and (3) psychological distress.

Conclusions. Our results add to the growing body of knowledge that emphasizes the negative health impacts of underregulated, high-risk, and physically demanding work performed primarily by im/migrants.

Public Health Implications. Our findings highlight the larger social–structural conditions and context of hardships endemic to migrant labor and suggest implications for practice and policy interventions.
(*Am J Public Health*. 2024;114(8):824–832. https://doi.org/10.2105/AJPH.2024.307696)

AJPH August 2024, Vol. 114, No. 8

Despite working in one of the most dangerous industries, commercial shrimp fishermen (shrimpers) are an understudied population.[1] In 2019, the fishing industry exhibited an occupational fatality rate nearly 40 times higher than the national average, which reflects hazardous working conditions, strenuous labor, long work hours, and harsh weather.[2] In the Gulf of Mexico, vessel disasters and falls overboard account for nearly 80% of fatalities, with nearly 50% of deaths occurring in the shellfish industry.[2] At any given time, there are approximately 23 000 commercial fishermen in the Gulf of Mexico, with a vast aging, low-socioeconomic-status (SES), and im/migrant population of workers.[3–5] Moreover, research shows that aging, low-SES, and im/migrant workers experience marginalization and precarity at higher rates than their counterparts.[6,7]

The disproportionately high number of fatalities among shrimpers in the Gulf of Mexico is a major concern for the field of public health, yet little is known about the contributing factors to injury among them. Surprisingly, there is limited qualitative empirical research on occupational safety, health, and well-being of shrimpers in the Gulf of Mexico.[8–11] The few existing studies are primarily quantitative and focus on safety trainings or health education.[8,10] Less known are whether cultural and interpersonal variables (social) as well as political and economic conditions (structural) are related to fatal and nonfatal events.

To address this research lacunae and to identify appropriate preventive interventions among Gulf of Mexico shrimpers, we conducted a qualitative study that examined the social–structural dimensions that contribute to health inequities. Specifically, we used participatory research methods to explore slips, trips, and falls among shrimpers, but we conceptualized injuries as detached neither from their individual choices nor from social–structural conditions. In this way, we examined power throughout our research as both a theoretical construct and an empirical question. Theoretically, we understood power as transactional—fluid and dynamic, both subtle and overt, and always-already connected to knowledge creation.[12] Empirically, we were interested in the health impacts of precarious and dangerous work that a higher proportion of im/migrants experience relative to non-im/migrant populations.[13] Overall, the team took a multifactorial approach to the research question, such as identifying social–structural determinants of health among the population and how they impacted their safety and health.

METHODS

We selected southeast Texas and the Rio Grande Valley (RGV) in Texas to examine shrimpers' potential hardships or obstacles to workplace safety between April 2021 and September 2022. We conducted semistructured interviews (n = 57; n = 26 in southeast Texas and n = 31 in RGV), 7 focus groups (n = 34), photovoice (n = 4 cameras returned; 2 interviews), and workplace observations with shrimpers to examine behaviors, risks, and everyday interactions (> 200 hours). In addition to identifying research questions from a multifactorial approach, our team also took a participatory approach to the study, which included partnerships between researchers, decision-makers, and participants. Partnerships included a shared responsibility for and contribution to the research. For example, we engaged with the fishing community on their terms, including spending time on the docks (to get to know people and build trust outside of official interviews) and providing health care and social services they requested (i.e., the Docside Clinic).[14] Participatory approaches have been increasingly recognized within public health as a necessary process for intentional, long-term research engagement with communities that places participants' needs, perspectives, and values at the center of research questions and interventions.[15,16]

Participants

Participants were recruited using snowball sampling and comprised 98% men and 2% women, 51% Vietnamese and 49% Latino; 30% experienced unstable housing; their average income ranged from $1000 to $6000 per trip (typically 30–45 days); and their ages ranged from 19 to 71 years. In the RGV, participants were mostly Mexican citizens using H-2B visas (a temporary, 6- to 9-month work visa that is not a pathway to residency status or citizenship), while in southeast Texas most participants were Vietnamese refugees. While many participants self-disclosed their visa or refugee status, citizenship status was purposefully not collected because of the numerous risks it poses for participants. The interviews were conducted by the principal investigator, research manager, and interpreter on the shrimp vessels or at the docks. Although the research team consisted of fluent Spanish- and Vietnamese-speaking members, an interpreter was also used to ensure that all interviews were conducted with someone who was a native Spanish or Vietnamese speaker trained in conducting interviews.

Data Collection and Photovoice Procedures

We followed a standardized informed consent protocol following institutional review board guidelines.[17] All participants were reassured that their responses were confidential such that boat owners, captains, or managers would not have access to responses, and participants received a $25 gift card for interviews or focus groups and a $50 gift card for photovoice. Observations included events where shrimpers meet and interact, both informal (e.g., the dock) and formal (e.g., fishery council meetings).[18–20]

The combination of traditional qualitative research methods with participatory approaches, like creating a health clinic with input from participants and photovoice, helped center the perspectives and experiences of shrimpers.[21,22] Historically, photovoice was developed as an avenue to have participants communicate what is important in their lives and from their perspectives instead of from the viewpoint of the researcher.[23] However, it has also evolved into a method that allows diverse audiences to see the lives of people whose work is often rendered invisible from public spaces.[24] We asked participants to take photos after we established a trusting relationship, and they participated in either an interview or focus group. The process we followed is consistent with photovoice literature that shows no relationship between group size and quality of participation; instead, long-term trust and rapport has a greater influence on the photos and interviews.[25] On average, shrimpers were given 1 month to take photographs. After they returned the cameras, we printed the photos and then brought them back to the docks and conducted interviews with the photographer-participant.

Data Analysis

We approached data analyses by using reflexive thematic analysis, which included emphasizing our own subjective experiences and knowledge as part of the analytical process.[14,26,27] This included the research team discussing our social identities and lived experiences, as well as our knowledge of extant research on im/migrant health or labor studies, and how these factors might influence the data analysis process. Theoretically, our methodical lens emphasized the importance and complexity of our social–structural positions, with a particular emphasis on how power is exercised as both repressive and disciplinary.[12]

The first stage of our analysis involved reading and rereading the semistructured interviews, focus group discussions, photovoice interviews, and field notes using a deductive approach to identify constructs based on previous theoretical orientations.[26] Constructs examined in the interviews included examining how power operates among shrimpers, the ways that structural violence appears in interpersonal and organizational relationships, and how social–structural dimensions of health impact individual injury. This approach allowed us to import our theoretical lens into the analysis process and explore contextual factors.

The second stage involved creating and assigning codes (i.e., short phrases to describe data) to meaningful text segments. Initially, each person read 1 transcript and assigned codes. The team then met to discuss the codes, reasons for coding in a particular way, and discrepancies. Codes were then created in Atlas.ti Cloud version 24 (ATLAS.ti Scientific Software Development GmbH, Berlin, Germany) by each researcher after we discussed our close reading of the data, but intercoder reliability was not calculated because the purpose of the analysis was not to ensure mutually agreed-upon interpretations of the data. That said, data were coded similarly with only minor differences, such as someone coding larger segments rather than smaller quotes or 2 people using interchangeable phrases (e.g., "sick leave" vs "benefits"). Only interview and focus group transcripts were coded, while field notes were used to provide context to our process.

The team managed the data within the Atlas.ti Cloud system, including assigning codes, creating code managers and groups, viewing code co-occurrences, and managing quotations. After coding was complete, the data were analyzed to explore themes related to fatal and nonfatal injury among shrimpers, but we analyzed their stories of injury through individual choices (e.g., not wearing a personal floatation device) as well as social–structural variables. Finally, after our analysis was complete, we conducted a follow-up focus group with a subset of shrimpers (n = 9) who had previously participated in an interview or focus group to share our findings or correct misinterpretations.

RESULTS

Multiple layers of vulnerability and danger exist among Gulf of Mexico shrimpers. In addition to vulnerabilities such as slips, trips, and falls, we found that social–structural factors are manifested through lack of access to health care and social needs. We interpreted the results from the interviews into 3 themes: (1) recognizing risk, (2) precarious employment, and (3) psychological distress.

Recognizing Risk

The first theme, recognizing risk, was born out of the many instances shrimpers described the deadly nature of their job (see Box 1). Shrimpers routinely identified falls overboard as a potential hazard or described in detail watching a crewmate fall overboard, but said matter-of-factly that these were the jobs immigrants have to get. Although slips, trips, and falls were common and frequently identified as a danger by shrimpers, they were quick to shift the focus away from these dangers, often justifying them with what could be seen as a fatalist attitude. Many other shrimpers understood the risk of slipping and falling overboard, but almost every person said they do not wear a personal flotation device (PFD). Overwhelmingly, they responded that it was uncomfortable to wear, difficult to work in because of its bulkiness, or too hot to wear in the summer. When asked what they would do to improve safety, conversations mostly turned to individual behaviors, like being smart and cautious of surroundings. However, there were some shrimpers who said boat owners also had a responsibility to maintain and replace broken equipment.

Shrimpers are not only calculating injuries but also the deadly risk from sharks that follow their boats for an easy meal (see Figure 1). Shrimpers often climb the trawls to fix various issues, and without a PFD, sharks are one more danger they face from slips, trips, and falls. Although the Coast Guard requires a life jacket on board for every person, it is not mandatory to wear it. Thus, shrimpers' use of

BOX 1— Participant Interview Data: Southeast and Rio Grande Valley, TX, April 2021–September 2022

Theme	Location and Job	Quote
Recognizing risk		
Falls overboard	Southeast Texas, Deckhand	"We never told anybody, but so many people die . . . so today, I'm going to tell you. . . . So many people died because of these hazards . . . nothing is safe here."
Safety	Rio Grande Valley, Deckhand	"A lot of people have fallen into the water, a lot of things have happened, but all jobs have risks, even in an office. This one is just a lot more, but this is the type of jobs the majority of immigrants have to get. That's just the way it is."
Wearing PFDs	Rio Grande Valley, Deckhand	"No, because it's [PFD] uncomfortable."
Wearing PFDs	Rio Grande Valley, Captain	"No. We don't use them [PFDs] because you can't do the maneuver with a vest on. And then we are carrying tools and you just can't. The vest, we wear when there is a lot of water coming into the boat or there is a storm but normally, we don't wear it."
Precarious employment		
Health care access	Southeast Texas, Former Deckhand	When a group of fishermen was asked about what services were available to help them when injured, one man replied, "Bud Light [beer]," to which others laughed in agreement.
Sick leave benefits	Rio Grande Valley, Deckhand	One Rio Grande Valley worker said, "I lost all my teeth in a crash. My nose was cut open and everything in my mouth. I didn't want to call the Coast Guard. The boss wanted me to return to land, but I need the money, I needed to work, so I put up with it at sea with pills for pain and infection to handle the trip."
Seasonal work	Southeast Texas, Captain	"They make a lot of money but one thing, they don't have no ID . . . they lost their IDs, green card, or whatever, I don't know, and they don't have no car, no transportation. They can't go nowhere. They're nice, they're good people, you know."
Seasonal work	Rio Grande Valley, Deckhand	"The only defect is that the visa is only given for 6–8 months . . . the government knows that we are coming to work and that we are not here to do anything bad. Our record is clean. We are not drinking. I wish the government would give us a longer visa so that we could work. Because then the visa expires, and we have to leave the country and go back to Mexico and look for work there and while they authorize us to work again and it's not easy to adapt there because what we know is how to fish and we have to look for a job in construction or something. We can't work at a business because it's for short periods of time. We have to wait until we get the next visa."
Psychological distress		
Loneliness	Rio Grande Valley, Deckhand	One shrimper likened the job to being in jail: "It's different for us because the majority of the time we are surrounded by and out in the water . . . it's as if you were in jail."
Loneliness	Rio Grande Valley, Deckhand	"It was difficult to get used to this way of life. Physically. Mentally. I think the biggest problem is in the head. The Americans say, you're homesick . . . because that's what hurts the most, we don't see our kids, we don't see our wives."
Loneliness	Rio Grande Valley, Deckhand	"Yes [it's hard on the family when you leave], even more for my little one, when he comes to say bye to me from where we leave, he starts crying . . . [he is] 6 years . . . it's tough. All your life at sea. Not seeing the kids grow up or anything."

Note. PFD = personal flotation device.

protective equipment is situated within complex calculations of risk based on lived experience, social norms, and weighing other hazards on the water.

Precarious Employment

Precarious employment is defined as insecure and unstable work that lacks social and economic benefits.[24] Shrimpers often described their work in these terms (see Box 1), which we categorized into 3 subthemes: health care options, sick leave benefits, and seasonal work.

Health care options. Shrimpers' lack of health care options varied, but included lack of coverage, little time to make appointments between shrimping trips, financial and language barriers, and lost, stolen, or incorrect citizenship documentation.[28] Most deck hands lacked primary health care, and their health care access was limited to emergency care. Participants routinely asked for medical supply kits for their vessels or an on-site clinic to address medical issues. A lack of health care options not only decreases preventive care but also leads to self-medication, such as an increase in substance use. Indeed, shrimpers often joked to us about their

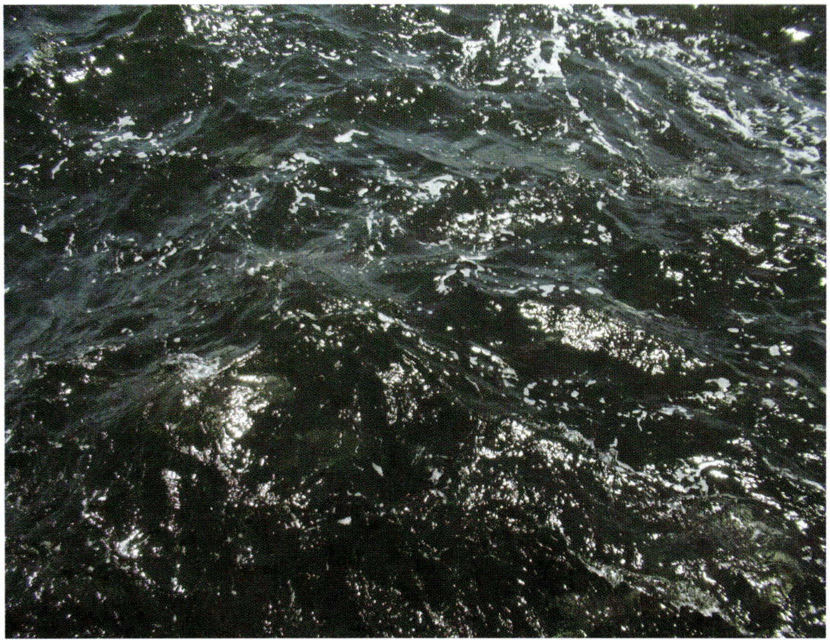

FIGURE 1— Photo of a Shark in the Water Taken by a Shrimper in the Gulf of Mexico

Note. When we asked one of the shrimpers in southeast Texas about the photos he took and if he was wearing a personal flotation device when leaning over the boat, he replied matter-of-factly, "No. There is nothing we can do in those." Another shrimper described the constant threat of sharks, and when asked if he feared them, responded with a laugh, "Yeah."

AJPH August 2024, Vol. 114, No. 8

substance use. Tellingly, nonfatal work-related injury is a leading cause of opioid misuse, self-medication, and overdose death, with higher prevalence of opioid use disorder in those with heavy physical jobs, more precarious work, and limited health care benefits, such as shrimpers.[29]

Sick leave benefits. In addition, social and economic factors, such as incentives to work while ill, contribute to increased health and safety risk. Workers reported that an absence of sick leave benefits influenced their health-seeking behaviors like delaying medical care and working while sick (see Figure 2).

Seasonal work. The seasonal and contractual nature of the work alongside citizenship documentation requirements created other restrictions for fishermen, such as the ability to apply for housing and government assistance. Housing insecurity, in particular, was a complicated issue. In southeast Texas, approximately one third of the non–H-2B Vietnamese refugees were living seasonally unhoused in broken down cars or in tents under elevated trailers, and participants routinely requested basic assistance with housing and food. In the RGV, where nearly half of the shrimpers are on H-2B visas, the employers are expected to provide or arrange housing,[30] but none of the H-2B workers we interviewed were receiving employer-sponsored housing. Most of the workers we spoke to in the RGV lived with family, crossed into Mexico, or paid for apartments out of pocket. One participant noted that an owner was building a dorm-style building for the workers, but at the time of the interviews, it was not yet ready, and the shrimpers were finding and paying for their own housing.

In the RGV, H-2B workers expressed their desire for the visa timeline to be extended, stating that the 8-month allowance was not enough time in the United States and that it was difficult to find a company in Mexico willing to hire them when they returned home. Thus, the rapid turnover and short timeframe between visa approval and visa expiration directly placed workers in a precarious position because it does not allow them to settle in and acquire resources to ensure well-being.

Psychological Distress

Finally, psychological distress and the lack of social and familial connection were prominent themes (see Box 1). Shrimpers' stories often centered on isolation, such as describing the loneliness of being at sea for 30 to 45 days at a time or not seeing their children. Interestingly, some shrimpers also described the beauty of being at sea or at the docks at sunset and sunrise,

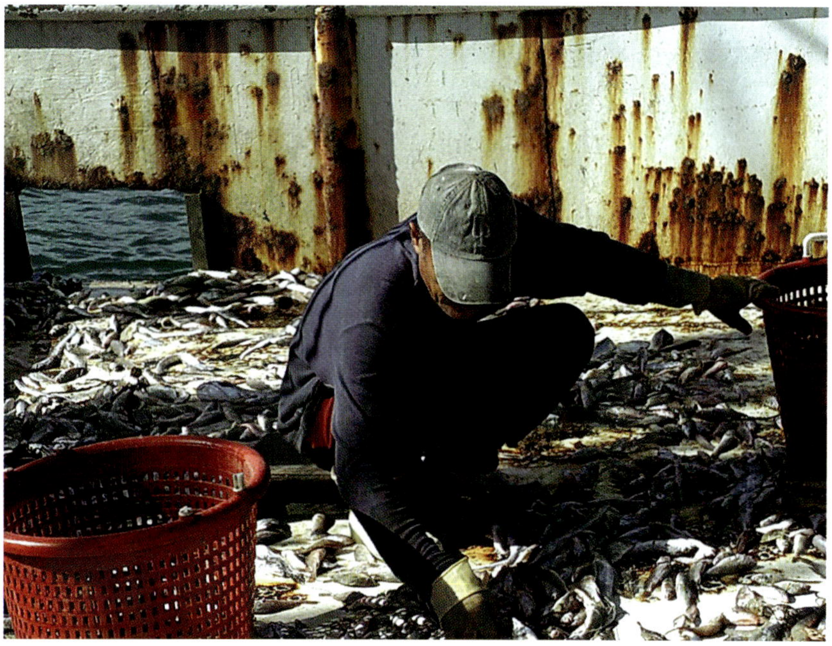

FIGURE 2— Photo of a Shrimper Working on the Boat Before He Was Injured

Note. A worker from southeast Texas who took this photo told us, "He [the man in the photo] got a seizure right after this picture, just before we finished this work. The whole net fell, and he hit his head and split his head from one side to another. Then he started seizing. He was trying to fix the holes in the net that were bitten by sharks. He is okay now." When asked what happened next, the interviewee responded that the man was flown off the boat by helicopter and spent 4 days in the hospital.

emphasizing the peace of solitude or the stars at night (see Figure 3). One shrimper, who lives seasonally unhoused at the docks, told us, "We don't have a 5-star hotel; we have the hotel of 10,000 stars." As we see through their experiences, perspectives of beauty coexist among loneliness. The shrimpers cannot be reduced to passive participants in these systems and openly discussed things they love about their work, but they also recognized that inequitable policies make this industry more dangerous for mainly im/migrant workers.

DISCUSSION

In the first participatory and qualitative research project, to our knowledge, among Gulf of Mexico shrimpers, we found that their injuries could not be delinked from their social–structural context. For example, behavioral health choices (e.g., self-medication to treat pain, not taking diabetes medication) were intimately connected to workers' lack of primary care access, which was linked to social–structural conditions like immigration status. Shrimpers appreciated the risk and danger associated with their work, but what can often be seen as a fatalist attitude or behavioral choice toward such risk can also be traced to their social position as im/migrants and how power operates or is diminished among certain populations. For instance, H-2B visa employers are expected and encouraged to provide workers with housing because of the difficulty of finding housing as a non–English-speaking migrant worker, yet none of the H-2B workers reported receiving housing assistance—one more example of how economic exploitation and power operate to create health inequity. Tellingly, danger and risk were not only caused by slips, trips, and falls, but also policies (e.g., shrimp import prices) that impact how much money a shrimper will make and, thus, how much they can reinvest in their boats or whether they can afford housing.[31] In this way, we see how shrimping is more dangerous because of a lack of social and regulatory (i.e., structural) policies that impact their physical and psychological health.

Therefore, the power fishermen have regarding their safety or housing was intimately steeped in social–structural conditions that grow out of neoliberalism, which is a political–economic theory focused on industry deregulation, decreased labor power, free enterprise, and personal responsibility that disciplines people to act in certain ways that may be against their best interests.[24,32] Neoliberalism becomes

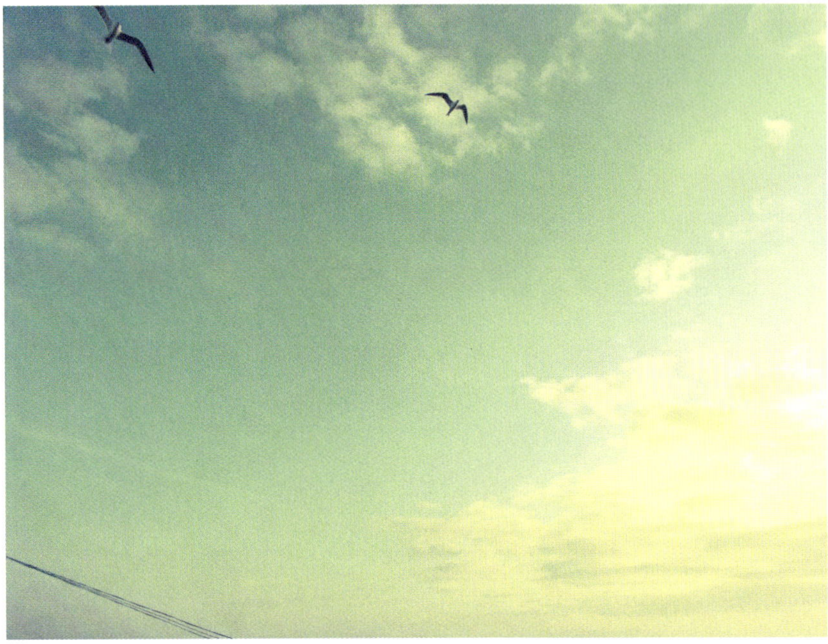

FIGURE 3— Photo of the Sky Taken by a Shrimper in the Gulf of Mexico

Note. The photovoice participant who took this photo, when asked why he took so many photos of the sky and birds, replied, "I found it peaceful out at sea."

AJPH August 2024, Vol. 114, No. 8

knowable and actionable not only through legislative policy (i.e., how power is operationalized as repressive) but also through the diffused discursive practices that produce subjects to a particular mode (i.e., how power is operationalized as disciplinary).[12,32] In the case of im/migrant shrimpers, they are not only expendable commodities of the state, or what Harvey calls "disposable people," but they have also been disciplined to act in certain ways that produce more precarity, such as not wearing a flotation device to work faster.[32] To unpack our findings through these conceptions of power, we examine how we can disrupt exploitative systems through (1) a research-to-practice intervention that was the idea of and implemented with the shrimpers and (2) research-to-policy approaches to dismantle social–structural barriers to health care access.

Public Health Implications

Research-to-practice. One approach to reducing inequities among shrimpers was a mobile clinic that our team implemented at the docks. The Docside Clinic, as it became known, has served more than 300 patients since July 2021 by providing access to services they requested. The clinic, which emerged as a result of our research and is funded by the National Institute for Occupational Safety and Health and the Southwest Center for Agricultural, Health, Injury Prevention, and Education was intended to be a 1-time event, but is now held once a month and is expanding to 2 other docks in the Gulf of Mexico. For the existing clinic, there is an on-call physician, resident, nurse practitioner, social worker, and medical student each month, plus our research team. Specific services shrimpers requested, which they mentioned during informal conversations as part of our participatory approach and captured in our field notes, included diabetes and blood pressure screenings, antibiotics, influenza kits, dental exams, and COVID-19, influenza, and tetanus vaccines, as well as food, socks, blankets, sun hats, sunscreen, and sun shirts. In addition to these requested services, we also offered occupational therapy, HIV and sexually transmitted infection testing, and podiatry services based on extant research of fishing industry needs. The clinic is an example of what can be created when we listen and respond to the needs of participants. Its genesis grew out of conversations with shrimpers and their continued requests and needs to have primary health care access.[28]

Although our team is proud of the Docside Clinic and the health care access it provides to shrimpers, we also must address what makes the clinic necessary in the first place: a complicated and expensive health care system in the United States with real or perceived barriers to entry for non–English-speaking im/migrants. Health care access, in this sense, is understood broadly from a social–structural dimensions of health lens to include everything from diabetes or cancer screenings to housing or food assistance (and how those issues interact with and impact each other). Primary health care, including physical, mental, and social health care needs, is complicated to access among im/migrant workers in the United States because of costs, language and cultural barriers, documentation requirements, not having employee-sponsored health insurance or sick leave benefits, fear of deportation, and antiimmigrant rhetoric.[13,33] However, the access issues that shrimpers faced were (and are) a result of policy choices. Systemic oppression does not simply appear, but is imagined and intentionally designed. In the case of shrimpers, from import prices to cheap labor, multiple and complex factors (e.g., economic exploitation, neoliberal ideals) create their health inequities.

Research-to-policy. Addressing access to health care among im/migrants in the United States is not a new phenomenon and has been reported on by researchers, journalists, advocates, and im/migrant patients,[13,33] but it is important to explicitly state that these social–structural factors will not be eliminated through a mobile clinic alone. We contend that a multipronged research-to-practice and -policy approach is more sustainable and equitable, which provides health care access to people who need it now (i.e., research-to-practice) while also working toward long-term policy change that addresses issues of exploitation and health care access (i.e., research-to-policy). Therefore, our approach involved not only providing clinical services in real time but also working directly with participants, policymakers, and other decision-makers. For example, we created policy briefs for staffers in state and federal offices about the fatality rates and health care access issues among im/migrant workers, participated in the US Department of Labor's listening sessions about needed changes to the temporary worker visa program, worked with union and labor-organizing representatives to address issues of cheap and dangerous labor, and met with legislative representatives and their staffers to find out how we can better provide information to them in ways that move evidence-informed research into policymaking.

Conclusions

Occupational health scholars in the Gulf of Mexico have increasingly shown how slips, trips, and falls are a major contributing factor to injury and death, yet the voices of shrimpers are lacking in terms of whether or how these injuries are seen as a crisis or local solutions to mitigate these inequities. Although we do not purport that our results can take all the varied and diverse experiences of shrimpers into account, we do maintain that a more critical public health approach is the first of many necessary steps in elevating the voices of people most impacted by policies by working to equalize knowledge production toward coproduced solutions.[16,34] Similarly, as much as we have tried to be unbiased, we know that our history, knowledge, and experiences are not disconnected from this work; we, like the shrimpers, are not immune to the ways power operates in our research. With that said, we took steps to ensure the experiences of shrimpers were centered by spending time outside of official interviews with them, both casually on the docks and through the Docside Clinic, as well as asking them to show us their work-worlds, which are often hidden from public view, through photovoice. The results contribute yet another case study regarding the health impacts of underregulated, high-risk, and physically demanding work performed primarily by im/migrants. These highlight the larger social–structural conditions and context of hardships endemic to migrant labor and suggest implications for practice and policy interventions. AJPH

ABOUT THE AUTHORS

Shannon Guillot-Wright and Lacy Davis are with The University of Texas Health Science Center at Houston School of Public Health. Linh Truong is with the Center for Violence Prevention, University of Texas Medical Branch, Galveston. Heide Castañeda is with the Department of Anthropology, University of South Florida, Tampa. Anabel Rodriguez is with the School of Public Health, Texas A&M University, College Station.

CORRESPONDENCE

Correspondence should be sent to Shannon Guillot-Wright, PhD, 1200 Pressler St, Houston, TX 77030 (e-mail: shannon.p.guillotwright@uth.tmc.edu). Reprints can be ordered at https://www.ajph.org by clicking the "Reprints" link.

PUBLICATION INFORMATION

Full Citation: Guillot-Wright S, Davis L, Truong L, Castañeda H, Rodriguez A. "The hotel of 10,000 stars": the impact of social-structural determinants of health among im/migrant shrimpers in the Gulf of Mexico. *Am J Public Health*. 2024;114(8):824–832.

Acceptance Date: April 9, 2024.

DOI: https://doi.org/10.2105/AJPH.2024.307696

ORCID iD:
Shannon Guillot-Wright https://orcid.org/0000-0001-9024-6722

CONTRIBUTORS

S. Guillot-Wright led the writing of the article and conceptualized and designed the study. L. Davis and L. Troung helped with data collection and analysis. H. Castañeda and A. Rodriguez provided theoretical context. All authors provided drafting and revision feedback and helped shape the research and article.

ACKNOWLEDGMENTS

Funding for this research was largely supported by the Southwest Center for Agricultural Health, Injury Prevention, and Education through cooperative agreement U54-OH007541 from the Centers for Disease Control and Prevention (CDC), National Institute for Occupational Safety and Health (NIOSH). Partial funding support was also provided by CDC/NIOSH (T42OH008421) at The University of Texas Health Science Center at Houston School of Public Health.

We are humbled and grateful to the many shrimpers who let us into their lives and to our hilarious and gracious interpreters, CucHuyen (Cecile) Roberts and Cuc Hoa Trieu. We also could not have carried out this work without the support and friendship of Vanessa Casanova, PhD, Jeff R. Temple, PhD, Jeffrey L. Levin, PhD, N. Miles Farr, PhD, and Martha Diaz, RN, as well as Amanda Wickman, Leonard Wang, Bibiana Toro Figueria, Nhu Nguyen, and Ellie Cherryhomes. We are grateful to the many volunteers who gave their time and resources, including Dean Wright and Bruce M. Guillot.

Note. The authors' views do not necessarily reflect the opinions of the CDC or the institutions with which the authors are affiliated.

CONFLICTS OF INTEREST

The authors have no conflicts of interest to declare.

HUMAN PARTICIPANT PROTECTION

The study was approved by the institutional review board at The University of Texas Medical Branch at Galveston and deemed exempt on March 25, 2021.

REFERENCES

1. Lincoln JM, Carruth A, Cherry D, Kincl L, Syron LN. Occupational health research in the commercial fishing industry. *J Agromed.* 2021;26(1): 28–30. https://doi.org/10.1080/1059924X.2021.1849494
2. Centers for Disease Control and Prevention, National Institute for Occupational Safety and Health. Commercial fishing safety—NIOSH workplace safety and health topic. 2023. Available at: https://www.cdc.gov/niosh/topics/fishing/gulfofmexicoregion.html. Accessed March 1, 2024.
3. Posadas B. Know more about the commercial fishermen in the Gulf of Mexico states. SeaGrant Mississippi-Alabama. 2018. Available at: https://masgc.org/news/article/know-more-about-the-commercial-fishermen-in-the-gulf-of-mexico-states. Accessed September 19, 2023.
4. Najarro I. Texas Gulf Coast fishing industry struggles after Harvey. *Seattle Times.* October 2, 2017. Available at: https://www.seattletimes.com/business/texas-gulf-coast-fishing-industry-struggles-after-harvey. Accessed September 19, 2023.
5. LSU Ag Center Research and Extension. Racial and ethnic groups in the Gulf of Mexico. 2012. Available at: https://www.lsuagcenter.com/NR/rdonlyres/D7BD2C54-F5A1-4592-ABE1-EC0CBEEC4680/90008/RR116racialandethnicgroupsinthegulfofmexicoregionv.pdf. Accessed September 19, 2023.
6. Flores Morales J. Aging and undocumented: the sociology of aging meets immigration status. *Sociol Compass.* 2021;15(4):e12859. https://doi.org/10.1111/soc4.12859
7. Grenier A, Hatzifilalithis S, Laliberte-Rudman D, Kobayashi K, Marier P, Phillipson C. Precarity and aging: a scoping review. *Gerontologist.* 2019;60(8): e620–e632. https://doi.org/10.1093/geront/gnz135.
8. Carruth AK, Levin JL, Gilmore K, et al. Cultural influences on safety and health education among Vietnamese fishermen. *J Agromed.* 2010;15(4): 375–385. https://doi.org/10.1080/1059924X.2010.513647
9. Levin JL, Gilmore K, Shepherd S, et al. Factors influencing safety among a group of commercial fishermen along the Texas Gulf Coast. *J Agromed.* 2010;15(4):363–374. https://doi.org/10.1080/1059924X.2010.509701
10. Levin JL, Gilmore K, Carruth A, et al. Helping Gulf shrimpers adopt safety measures: importance of partnerships and research to practice. *J Agromed.* 2012;17(1):15–21. https://doi.org/10.1080/1059924X.2012.627312
11. Carruth AK, Levin JL. Cultural influences on safety training among Vietnamese shrimp fisherman. *J Agromed.* 2014;19(2):207–208. https://doi.org/10.1080/1059924X.2014.889624.
12. Foucault M. *Power/Knowledge: Selected Interviews and Other Writings, 1972–1977.* New York, NY: Pantheon Books; 1980.
13. Guillot-Wright S, Cherryhomes E, Wang L, Overcash M. Systems and subversion: a review of structural violence and im/migrant health. *Curr Opin Psychol.* 2022;47:101431. https://doi.org/10.1016/j.copsyc.2022.101431
14. Aléx L, Hammarström A. Shift in power during an interview situation: methodological reflections inspired by Foucault and Bourdieu. *Nurs Inq.* 2008; 15(2):169–176. https://doi.org/10.1111/j.1440-1800.2008.00398.x
15. Minkler M, Blackwell AG, Thompson M, Tamir H. Community-based participatory research: implications for public health funding. *Am J Public Health.* 2003;93(8):1210–1213. https://doi.org/10.2105/AJPH.93.8.1210
16. Bowleg L. Perspectives from the social sciences: critically engage public health. *Am J Public Health.* 2018;109(1):15–16. https://doi.org/10.2105/AJPH.2018.304825
17. Kaiser K. Protecting respondent confidentiality in qualitative research. *Qual Health Res.* 2009;19(11): 1632–1641. https://doi.org/10.1177/1049732309350879
18. Davies CA. *Reflexive Ethnography: A Guide to Researching Selves and Others.* 2007. Available at: https://www.routledge.com/Reflexive-Ethnography-A-Guide-to-Researching-Selves-and-Others/Davies-Davies/p/book/9780415409018. Accessed September 19, 2023.
19. Copland F, Creese A. *Linguistic Ethnography: Collecting, Analysing and Presenting Data.* SAGE Publications Ltd. 2015. Available at: https://methods.sagepub.com/book/linguistic-ethnography. Accessed September 19, 2023.
20. DeJonckheere M, Vaughn LM. Semistructured interviewing in primary care research: a balance of relationship and rigour. *Fam Med Community Health.* 2019;7(2):000057. https://doi.org/10.1136/fmch-2018-000057
21. Sutton-Brown CA. Photovoice: a methodological guide. *Photogr Cult.* 2015;7(2):169–185. https://doi.org/10.2752/175145214X13999922103165
22. Bourgois P, Schonberg J. *Righteous Dopefiend.* 1st ed. University of California Press. 2009. Available at: https://www.ucpress.edu/book/9780520254985/righteous-dopefiend. Accessed September 19, 2023.
23. Wang C, Burris MA. Photovoice: concept, methodology, and use for participatory needs assessment. *Health Educ Behav.* 1997;24(3):369–387. https://doi.org/10.1177/109019819702400309
24. Guillot-Wright S. "The company will fire you because you are too expensive": a photo-ethnography of health care rights among Filipino migrant seafarers. *Humanit Soc Sci Commun.* 2021;8(1):1–10. https://doi.org/10.1057/s41599-021-00947-y
25. Catalani C, Minkler M. Photovoice: a review of the literature in health and public health. *Health Educ Behav.* 2010;37(3):424–451. https://doi.org/10.1177/1090198109342084
26. Braun V, Clarke V. One size fits all? What counts as quality practice in (reflexive) thematic analysis? *Qual Res Psychol.* 2020;18(3):328–352. https://doi.org/10.1080/14780887.2020.1769238
27. Braun V, Clarke V. Reflecting on reflexive thematic analysis. *Qual Res Sport Exerc Health.* 2019;11(4): 589–597. https://doi.org/10.1080/2159676X.2019.1628806
28. Guillot-Wright S, Farr NM, Cherryhomes E. A community-led mobile health clinic to improve structural and social determinants of health among (im)migrant workers. *Int J Equity Health.* 2022;21(1):58. https://doi.org/10.1186/s12939-022-01630-7
29. Walter AW, Morocho C, King L, et al. Preventing opioid use disorders among fishing industry workers. *Int J Environ Res Public Health.* 2018; 15(4):648. https://doi.org/10.3390/ijerph15040648
30. Harris Beach PLLC Attorneys at Law. It's H-2B Visa season: what seasonal employers need to know for 2022. Available at: https://www.harrisbeach.com/insights/its-h-2b-visa-season-what-seasonal-employers-need-to-know-for-2022. Accessed March 1, 2024.
31. Guillot-Wright S. The changing economic structure of the maritime industry and its adverse effects on seafarers' health care rights. *Int Marit Health.* 2017;68(2):77–82. https://doi.org/10.5603/IMH.2017.0015
32. Harvey D. *A Brief History of Neoliberalism.* Oxford, England: Oxford University Press; 2005. https://doi.org/10.1093/oso/9780199283262.001.0001
33. Rodriguez A, Lopez SN, Douphrate DI. On-farm health screening needs of immigrant dairy workers in the Texas Panhandle and South Plains. *J Agromed.* 2023;28(4):665–675. https://doi.org/10.1080/1059924X.2023.2200418
34. Schrecker T. What is critical about critical public health? Focus on health inequalities. *Crit Public Health.* 2021;32(2):139–144. https://doi.org/10.1080/09581596.2021.1905776

Preexposure Prophylaxis (PrEP) for HIV Prevention at Outpatient Substance Use Treatment Facilities, United States, 2021

Samuel R. Bunting, MD, MSHA, Nitin Vidyasagar, BS, Allison P. Wilson, BA, and Aniruddha Hazra, MD

Objectives. To determine the percentage of US outpatient substance use treatment facilities that offer HIV preexposure prophylaxis (PrEP).

Methods. We used a retrospective cross-sectional design with data from the National Substance Use and Mental Health Services Survey, which was administered to directors of US outpatient substance use treatment facilities in 2021. We evaluated the percentage of outpatient substance use treatment facilities offering PrEP and factors associated with the likelihood of offering PrEP.

Results. We included 12 182 outpatient substance use treatment facilities. Of these, 637 (5.2%) offered PrEP. Offering HIV treatment (adjusted odds ratio [AOR] = 45.3; 95% confidence interval [CI] = 36.0, 56.9) and offering programs for LGBTQ (lesbian, gay, bisexual, transgender, and queer or questioning) people (AOR = 1.3; 95% CI = 1.0, 1.6) were associated with higher likelihoods of offering PrEP.

Conclusions. PrEP is highly effective and recommended for patients at risk for HIV from injection drug use. Nearly 95% of US outpatient substance use treatment facilities did not offer PrEP—a missed opportunity for harm reduction through primary HIV prevention.

Public Health Implications. Diversification of the array of available HIV PrEP options and the ongoing HIV and opioid use epidemics require outpatient substance use treatment facilities to expand PrEP availability. (*Am J Public Health*. 2024;114(8):833–837. https://doi.org/10.2105/AJPH.2024.307699)

AJPH August 2024, Vol. 114, No. 8

The US Centers for Disease Control and Prevention (CDC) reported more than 36 000 new HIV diagnoses in 2021, including more than 2500 attributed to intravenous drug use.[1] People with substance use disorders (SUD) experience a disproportionate incidence of HIV, and there are periodic clusters of HIV cases among people who inject drugs (PWID).[2,3] This disproportionate incidence is occurring in the context of the ongoing US opioid epidemic.

Daily antiretroviral preexposure prophylaxis (PrEP) with emtricitabine/tenofovir disoproxil fumarate is up to 99% effective in preventing HIV transmission via sexual contact and 74% effective via intravenous drug use.[4] The US Preventive Service Task Force for PWID recommends HIV PrEP.[5] Despite this documented efficacy and recommendation, uptake of PrEP among people with SUD, including PWID, remains low.[6] Recent work estimated that only 0.15% of PWID were prescribed PrEP.[6]

The federal Ending the HIV Epidemic policy framework and the National HIV/AIDS Strategy both place specific emphasis on the integration of PrEP and HIV prevention services through integrated care models uniquely designed for hard-to-reach patient populations, including people with SUD and PWID, who are vulnerable to contracting HIV.[7,8] Previous work has demonstrated an increase in HIV testing in substance use treatment facilities following the beginning of the HIV epidemic, with up to 86% providing testing in 2000.[9,10] However, a recent study found that only 29% of outpatient substance use treatment facilities offered HIV testing in 2018.[11]

The integration of PrEP prescriptions into substance use treatment facilities, an important step in the HIV prevention care continuum, has been less studied. A previous intervention in an opioid use clinic found that less than a third of patients with opioid use disorder (OUD) were aware of PrEP and that none were taking PrEP despite HIV vulnerability from sexual encounters or intravenous drug use.[12] A second intervention, focused exclusively on PWID experiencing homelessness, found high PrEP interest but also high discontinuation rates, reinforcing the need for sustainable services in easily accessible care settings.[13] We examined HIV PrEP implementation in outpatient substance use care settings with a large national data set.

METHODS

This was a retrospective, cross-sectional analysis of existing, publicly available, administrative data collected through the National Substance Use and Mental Health Services Survey (N-SUMHSS), which is administered by the Substance Abuse and Mental Health Services Administration (SAMHSA).[14] The N-SUMHSS is distributed to all known inpatient and outpatient mental health and substance use treatment facilities in the United States and Puerto Rico. SAMHSA collected data online between April 2021 and January 2022.

The primary outcome for this study was whether facilities offered PrEP, phrased on the N-SUMHSS as medications for preexposure prophylaxis (e.g., emtricitabine/tenofovir disoproxil fumarate combination, and emtricitabine and tenofovir alafenamide combination). Available responses were yes and no. We included additional N-SUMHSS items to describe facility characteristics, including primary focus, ownership, accepted insurance, federal OUD treatment certification, US state (collapsed into region), whether offering medication for OUD, specific services for lesbian, gay, bisexual, transgender, and queer or questioning (LGBTQ) patients with SUD, whether offering medications for HIV treatment, and whether offering long-acting injectable (LAI)-buprenorphine.

We calculated frequencies to describe the percentage and characteristics of facilities that offered PrEP. We conducted multivariable binomial logistic regression to evaluate the combined effects of facility characteristics on the likelihood of offering PrEP. Finally, we calculated the Spearman rho to evaluate correlation between the HIV diagnosis rate in a state, taken from the CDC, and the percentage of outpatient substance use facilities offering PrEP.[1] We analyzed the data using Stata/MP version 17 (StataCorp, College Station, TX), and we followed Strengthening the Reporting of Observational Studies in Epidemiology reporting guidelines.

RESULTS

The 2021 N-SUMHSS was sent to 28 298 facilities and had a response rate of 78.8%.[14] We restricted the data set to facilities that indicated that they offered outpatient substance use treatment services and that did not have any missing data for any of the variables of interest (n = 12 182). Full descriptive information of the included facilities is provided in Table 1, and sample restriction is presented in Figure A (available as a supplement to the online version of this article at http://www.ajph.org).

Overall, 637 (5.2%) outpatient substance use facilities offered HIV PrEP. Facilities that offered any medication for OUD were more likely to offer PrEP (adjusted odds ratio [AOR] = 5.2; 95% confidence interval [CI] = 3.5, 7.9) as were those that offered HIV treatment (AOR = 45.3; 95% CI = 36.0, 56.9). Having services specific for LGBTQ clients was also associated with higher odds of offering PrEP (AOR = 1.3; 95% CI = 1.0, 1.6; Table 1). A total of 1018 facilities offered HIV treatment; 498 (48.9%) of these offered PrEP, and 520 did not. There were 2227 facilities (18.3%) that offered LAI-buprenorphine, and of these 328 (14.7%) offered PrEP. The correlation between state HIV diagnosis rate and the percentage of outpatient substance use treatment facilities offering PrEP in 2021 (Figure B, available as a supplement to the online version of this article at http://www.ajph.org) was not significant ($r = 0.16$; $P = .27$).

DISCUSSION

The ongoing opioid epidemic in the United States demands harm reduction efforts in addition to development and scaling treatments for OUD. Fentanyl has become a driver of the opioid epidemic, and this drug's short half-life requires more frequent injection, increasing vulnerability to HIV through needle sharing.[15–17] PrEP is an effective harm reduction intervention for people with SUD, including PWID; however, nearly 95% of outpatient substance use treatment facilities in the United States have not implemented PrEP—a critical missed opportunity for vulnerable and hard-to-reach patients. The lack of a

TABLE 1— Facility Characteristics Associated With Offering Preexposure Prophylaxis (PrEP): United States, 2021

	Facility Characteristics, No. (%)	Offer PrEP, No. (%)	Bivariate OR (95% CI)	Multivariable AOR (95% CI)
Service focus				
Substance use treatment	4368 (35.9)	103 (2.4)	1 (Ref)	1 (Ref)
Mental health services	854 (7.0)	40 (4.7)	2.0 (1.4, 3.0)	1.5 (1.0, 2.5)
Mix mental health and substance use treatment	6960 (57.1)	494 (7.1)	3.2 (2.6, 3.9)	1.7 (1.3, 2.3)
Ownership				
Private for-profit organization	5499 (39.5)	129 (2.7)	1 (Ref)	1 (Ref)
Private nonprofit organization	6729 (48.4)	311 (5.2)	2.0 (1.6, 2.5)	1.9 (1.4, 2.5)
State/local/federal/Tribal government	1678 (12.1)	197 (13.8)	5.8 (4.6, 7.3)	1.9 (1.4, 2.6)
Federally certified OUD treatment center				
No	10561 (86.7)	549 (5.2)	1 (Ref)	1 (Ref)
Yes	1621 (13.3)	88 (5.4)	1.1 (0.8, 1.3)	0.8 (0.6, 1.2)
Any medications for OUD				
No	5189 (42.6)	29 (0.6)	1 (Ref)	1 (Ref)
Yes	6993 (57.4)	608 (8.7)	16.9 (11.7, 24.6)	5.2 (3.5, 7.9)
Only treats OUD				
No	11096 (91.1)	620 (5.6)	1 (Ref)	1 (Ref)
Yes	1086 (8.9)	17 (1.6)	0.3 (0.2, 0.4)	0.5 (0.3, 0.9)
Affiliated with religious organization				
No	11697 (96.0)	611 (5.2)	1 (Ref)	1 (Ref)
Yes	485 (4.0)	26 (5.4)	1.0 (0.7, 1.5)	0.8 (0.5, 1.4)
Accepts Medicaid				
No	2559 (21.0)	171 (6.7)	1 (Ref)	1 (Ref)
Yes	9623 (79.0)	466 (4.8)	0.7 (0.6, 0.9)	1.0 (0.7, 1.3)
Accepts Medicare				
No	5688 (46.7)	206 (3.6)	1 (Ref)	1 (Ref)
Yes	6494 (53.3)	431 (6.6)	1.9 (1.6, 2.2)	1.5 (1.1, 2.0)
Accepts private insurance				
No	2619 (21.5)	97 (3.7)	1 (Ref)	1 (Ref)
Yes	9563 (78.5)	540 (5.7)	1.6 (1.3, 1.9)	0.9 (0.6, 1.2)
Region				
Northeast	2272 (18.7)	136 (6.0)	1 (Ref)	1 (Ref)
Midwest	3187 (26.2)	167 (5.2)	0.9 (0.7, 1.1)	1.0 (0.7, 1.3)
South	3670 (30.1)	182 (5.0)	0.8 (0.7, 1.0)	1.0 (0.8, 1.4)
West	3053 (25.1)	152 (5.0)	0.8 (0.7, 1.0)	1.1 (0.8, 1.5)
LGBTQ specific				
No	8417 (69.1)	382 (4.5)	1 (Ref)	1 (Ref)
Yes	3765 (30.9)	255 (6.8)	1.5 (1.3, 1.8)	1.3 (1.0, 1.6)
Offers HIV treatment				
No	11164 (91.6)	139 (1.3)	1 (Ref)	1 (Ref)
Yes	1018 (8.4)	498 (48.9)	76.0 (61.7, 93.5)	45.3 (36.0, 56.9)

Note. AOR = adjusted odds ratio; CI = confidence interval; LGBTQ = lesbian, gay, bisexual, transgender, queer or questioning; OR = odds ratio; OUD = opioid use disorder. The percentages of facilities in each group offering PrEP represent the percentage of facilities in each category in the far left column that indicated offering PrEP to patients. Bivariate ORs represent the bivariate logistic regressions, and AORs represent the multivariable analyses adjusting for the effects of all covariates.

significant correlation between the state-level percentage of facilities offering PrEP and the HIV diagnosis rate also suggests a lack of response to public health needs.

A previous study of outpatient substance use treatment facilities found that community need and context (e.g., high percentage of underserved patients) were significant predictors of offering HIV testing, suggesting that a similar response for scaling PrEP availability may be possible.[9] However, previous research indicates that most PWID remain unaware of PrEP; for example, a 2020 qualitative study found that more than two thirds of interviewed PWID were unaware of PrEP.[18] When queried for PrEP interest, PWID were found to be highly interested in taking PrEP, yet they were faced with logistical, clinical, and structural barriers to accessing it (e.g., housing instability, lack of transportation, lack of clinic access, stigma).[18–20] These barriers likely contribute to the finding that less than 1% of PWID with private insurance were prescribed PrEP.[6] Interventions to colocate PrEP services in substance use treatment settings may minimize logistical barriers and improve the uptake of this effective prevention regimen.[12]

Encouragingly, facilities providing any medication for OUD were more likely to offer PrEP, suggesting a degree of colocation of harm reduction strategies in treating and preventing opioid use relapse and primary HIV prevention. Finally, approximately one fifth of outpatient substance use treatment facilities offered LAI-buprenorphine for OUD treatment, but only 14.7% also offered PrEP. With the December 2021 approval of LAI-cabotegravir for PrEP, these facilities may serve as outlets for scaling availability of LAI PrEP options in service models where LAI drugs (e.g., antipsychotics, LAI-buprenorphine, LAI-naltrexone) are already provided.

Moreover, facilities offering HIV treatment without PrEP could quickly close this gap as the necessary clinical expertise and infrastructure for prescribing antiretrovirals and routine lab monitoring are likely already in place. Finally, we also found that facilities with a specific program for LGBTQ patients had slightly higher odds of offering PrEP. This is encouraging, considering the disproportionate incidence of HIV among LGBTQ populations, especially men who have sex with men,[1] and these programs may also serve as a model for scaling PrEP to all patients vulnerable to HIV.

Models such as the STI Express Initiative may also be rapidly adaptable to improving the availability of PrEP services at outpatient substance use facilities with minimal resource and staff requirements. Such models rely on peer educators and clinic staff guiding patients through self-testing for sexually transmitted infections and HIV and have been adapted to include same-day PrEP initiation.[21] Substance use treatment facilities are essential providers of harm reduction–focused care and care coordination, especially in rural areas; thus, expansion of PrEP availability is vital to ending the syndemic of HIV transmission amid the opioid epidemic.

Limitations

The findings of this study should be interpreted in the context of several limitations. First are the inherent limitations of cross-sectional survey data that represent a single point in time. Recall bias is also a possible limitation, and respondents may have answered survey items incorrectly. The wording of the PrEP item on the N-SUMHSS is also a possible limitation, as the question did not specifically inquire about HIV PrEP. However, the survey item did include the names of the only 2 oral antiretroviral medications that are approved for use as PrEP in the United States, reducing the possibility of a misunderstanding.

Finally, the number of facilities included in the total sample was limited because of missing data on the primary variables of interest. A more targeted study is needed to expand on the foundational results of this study and to assess for trends in the implementation of HIV PrEP as the HIV and OUD syndemics continue to evolve in the United States.

Conclusions

Ending the HIV epidemic in the United States requires all communities to have access to treatment and prevention. People with SUD, and specifically PWID, are a priority population for such targeted interventions. Outpatient SUD treatment facilities already provide community-informed services for the care of persons using drugs; this research identifies a major opportunity to expand their services to easily integrate HIV prevention.

Public Health Implications

The diversification of the array of available HIV PrEP options as well as the ongoing HIV and opioid use epidemics require outpatient substance use treatment facilities to expand availability of PrEP. AJPH

ABOUT THE AUTHORS

Samuel Bunting is with the Department of Psychiatry and Behavioral Neuroscience, University of Chicago, Chicago, IL. Nitin Vidyasagar is with the Pritzker School of Medicine, University of Chicago.

Allison Wilson and Aniruddha Hazra are with the Chicago Center for HIV Elimination, University of Chicago. Aniruddha Hazra is also with the Section of Infectious Diseases, Department of Medicine, University of Chicago.

CORRESPONDENCE

Correspondence should be sent to Samuel R. Bunting, MD, MSHA, Department of Psychiatry and Behavioral Neuroscience, University of Chicago, 5841 S. Maryland Ave, MC 3077, Chicago, IL 60637 (e-mail: Samuel.Bunting@bsd.uchicago.edu). Reprints can be ordered at https://www.ajph.org by clicking the "Reprints" link.

PUBLICATION INFORMATION

Full Citation: Bunting SR, Vidyasagar N, Wilson AP, Hazra A. Preexposure prophylaxis (PrEP) for HIV prevention at outpatient substance use treatment facilities, United States, 2021. *Am J Public Health*. 2024;114(8):833–837.

Acceptance Date: April 15, 2024.

DOI: https://doi.org/10.2105/AJPH.2024.307699

CONTRIBUTORS

S. R. Bunting conceptualized and designed the study, analyzed and interpreted the data, and provided study materials. S. R. Bunting and N. Vidyasagar collected and assembled the data. S. R. Bunting, N. Vidyasagar, and A. P. Wilson drafted the article. A. Hazra critically revised the article for important intellectual content and provided administrative, technical, and logistic support. All authors approved the final version of the article for publication.

CONFLICTS OF INTEREST

S. R. Bunting and A. Hazra received unrestricted research funding from Gilead Sciences for research unrelated to this study. S. R. Bunting reports support from the National Institute of Mental Health (5R25MH083620; Principal Investigator: Nunn). N. Vidyasagar and A. P. Wilson have no conflicts of interest to disclose.

HUMAN PARTICIPANT PROTECTION

The University of Chicago institutional review board determined this study to be non–human participant research and exempted it from review.

REFERENCES

1. Centers for Disease Control and Prevention. Diagnoses of HIV infection in the United States and dependent areas, 2021. May 23, 2023. Available at: https://www.cdc.gov/hiv/library/reports/hiv-surveillance/vol-34/index.html. Accessed April 29, 2024.
2. Lerner AM, Fauci AS. Opioid injection in rural areas of the United States: a potential obstacle to ending the HIV epidemic. *JAMA*. 2019;322(11):1041–1042. https://doi.org/10.1001/jama.2019.10657
3. Randall LM, Dasgupta S, Day J, et al. An outbreak of HIV infection among people who inject drugs in northeastern Massachusetts: findings and lessons learned from a medical record review. *BMC Public Health*. 2022;22(1):257. [Erratum in: *BMC Public Health*. 2022;22(1):412]. https://doi.org/10.1186/s12889-022-12604-3
4. Choopanya K, Martin M, Suntharasamai P, et al. Antiretroviral prophylaxis for HIV infection in injecting drug users in Bangkok, Thailand (the Bangkok Tenofovir Study): a randomised, double-blind, placebo-controlled phase 3 trial. *Lancet*. 2013;381(9883):2083–2090. https://doi.org/10.1016/S0140-6736(13)61127-7
5. US Preventive Services Task Force. Preexposure prophylaxis for the prevention of HIV infection: US Preventive Services Task Force recommendation statement. *JAMA*. 2019;321(22):2203–2213. https://doi.org/10.1001/jama.2019.6390
6. Streed CG Jr, Morgan JR, Gai MJ, Larochelle MR, Paasche-Orlow MK, Taylor JL. Prevalence of HIV preexposure prophylaxis prescribing among persons with commercial insurance and likely injection drug use. *JAMA Netw Open*. 2022;5(7):e2221346. https://doi.org/10.1001/jamanetworkopen.2022.21346
7. Das S, Muhetaer K, Alvarado HA. Changes in integrated HIV care in substance use treatment facilities (2015–2020). May 2, 2022. Available at: https://www.samhsa.gov/data/sites/default/files/Changes_in_inte_15.pdf. Accessed April 29, 2024.
8. Fauci AS, Redfield RR, Sigounas G, Weahkee MD, Giroir BP. Ending the HIV epidemic: a plan for the United States. *JAMA*. 2019;321(9):844–845. https://doi.org/10.1001/jama.2019.1343
9. Broffman L, D'Aunno T, Chang JE. Factors associated with the adoption of evidence-based innovations by substance use disorder treatment organizations: a study of HIV testing. *J Subst Abuse Treat*. 2023;144:108929. https://doi.org/10.1016/j.jsat.2022.108929
10. Pollack HA, D'Aunno T, Lamar B. Outpatient substance abuse treatment and HIV prevention: an update. *J Subst Abuse Treat*. 2006;30(1):39–47. https://doi.org/10.1016/j.jsat.2005.09.002
11. Riano NS, Borowsky HM, Arnold EA, et al. HIV testing and counseling at US substance use treatment facilities: a missed opportunity for early identification. *Psychiatr Serv*. 2021;72(12):1385–1391. https://doi.org/10.1176/appi.ps.202000524
12. Johnson J, Gormley MA, Bentley S, et al. HIV preexposure prophylaxis care continuum among individuals receiving medication for opioid use disorder, South Carolina, 2020–2021. *Am J Public Health*. 2022;112(1):34–37. https://doi.org/10.2105/AJPH.2021.306566
13. Biello KB, Bazzi AR, Vahey S, Harris M, Shaw L, Brody J. Delivering preexposure prophylaxis to people who use drugs and experience homelessness, Boston, MA, 2018–2020. *Am J Public Health*. 2021;111(6):1045–1048. https://doi.org/10.2105/AJPH.2021.306208
14. Substance Abuse and Mental Health Services Administration. National Substance Use and Mental Health Services Survey (N-SUMHSS). 2023. Available at: https://www.datafiles.samhsa.gov/dataset/national-substance-use-and-mental-health-services-survey-2021-n-sumhss-2021-ds0001. Accessed May 6, 2023.
15. Centers for Disease Control and Prevention. Opioid overdose. 2023. Available at: https://www.cdc.gov/drugoverdose/deaths/opioid-overdose.html. Accessed October, 2023.
16. Lambdin BH, Bluthenthal RN, Zibbell JE, Wenger L, Simpson K, Kral AH. Associations between perceived illicit fentanyl use and infectious disease risks among people who inject drugs. *Int J Drug Policy*. 2019;74:299–304. https://doi.org/10.1016/j.drugpo.2019.10.004
17. Alpren C, Dawson EL, John B, et al. Opioid use fueling HIV transmission in an urban setting: an outbreak of HIV infection among people who inject drugs—Massachusetts, 2015–2018. *Am J Public Health*. 2020;110(1):37–44. https://doi.org/10.2105/AJPH.2019.305366
18. Allen ST, O'Rourke A, White RH, et al. Barriers and facilitators to PrEP use among people who inject drugs in rural Appalachia: a qualitative study. *AIDS Behav*. 2020;24(6):1942–1950. https://doi.org/10.1007/s10461-019-02767-3
19. Biello KB, Bazzi AR, Mimiaga MJ, et al. Perspectives on HIV pre-exposure prophylaxis (PrEP) utilization and related intervention needs among people who inject drugs. *Harm Reduct J*. 2018;15(1):55. https://doi.org/10.1186/s12954-018-0263-5
20. Sherman SG, Schneider KE, Park JN, et al. PrEP awareness, eligibility, and interest among people who inject drugs in Baltimore, Maryland. *Drug Alcohol Depend*. 2019;195:148–155. https://doi.org/10.1016/j.drugalcdep.2018.08.014
21. National Association of County and City Health Officials. Implementing express STI services: considerations and lessons learned. 2021. Available at: https://www.naccho.org/uploads/downloadable-resources/Implementing-Express-STI-Services-Guide.pdf. Accessed April 29, 2024.

Erratum In: "Rapid Community Translation in the Colorado CEAL (CO-CEAL) Program: Transcreating Messaging to Promote COVID-19 Vaccination"

In: Brewer SE, Fisher M, Zittleman L, et al. Rapid community translation in the Colorado CEAL (CO-CEAL) program: transcreating messaging to promote COVID-19 vaccination. *Am J Public Health*. 2024;114(S1):S50–S54.

When originally published, author Amanda Skenadore's last name was listed incorrectly in the article byline and in the "About the Authors" section. On p. S50, their name in the article byline should read: "Amanda Skenadore, MPH." On p. S53 in the "About the Authors" section, the fourth to last sentence should read: "Amanda Skenadore is with ACCORDS."

These changes do not affect the article's conclusions. AJPH

https://doi.org/10.2105/AJPH.2023.307456e

Erratum In: "Retention of Community Health Workers in the Public Health Workforce: Public Health Workforce Interests and Needs Survey, 2017 and 2021"

In: Kirkland C, Dill JS, Karnik H. Retention of community health workers in the public health workforce: Public Health Workforce Interests and Needs Survey, 2017 and 2021. *Am J Public Health*. 2024;114(1):44–47.

When originally published, the Figure 1 key incorrectly listed the bar color identifiers. On p. 45, the key should identify the white bars as representative of "Dissatisfied" community health workers and the gray bars as representative of "Satisfied/Neutral" community health workers.

On p. 45, Figure 1 should appear as:

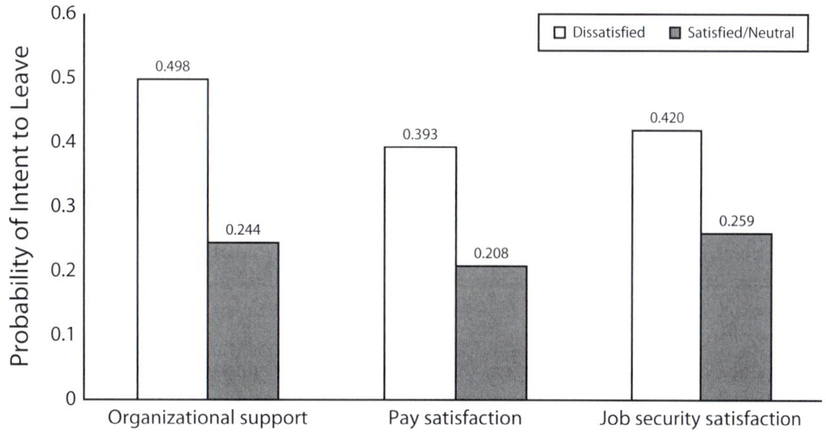

FIGURE 1— Percentage Likelihood That CHWs Will Indicate an Intent to Leave Their Position on the Basis of Experienced Organizational Support, Pay Satisfaction, and Job Security Satisfaction: United States, 2017 and 2021

Note. CHW = community health worker. There were 806 observations; the estimated population size was 3893.

This change does not affect the article's conclusions. AJPH

https://doi.org/10.2105/AJPH.2023.307462e

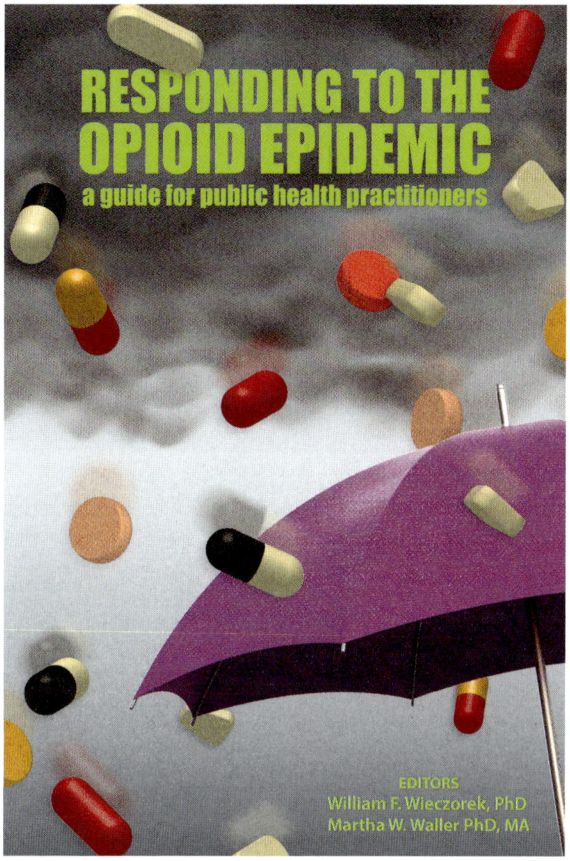

ISBN 978-0-87553-344-5, 400 PP., 2024,
SOFTBOUND/PRINT-ON-DEMAND

Responding to the Opioid Epidemic: A Guide for Public Health Practitioners

Edited by: William F. Wieczorek, PhD and Martha W. Waller PhD, MA

It's impossible to completely prevent the substance misuse defining the opioid epidemic, and it's impossible to treat the problem away. This reality requires a continuum of care (COC) approach, which includes promotion, prevention, case-finding, treatment, and recovery. This book presents research-informed interventions aligned with the COC approach to guide how communities, first responders, lay persons, medical providers, policymakers, treatment providers, and others can respond to the opioid epidemic at an individual, community, state, and national level.

APHABOOKSTORE.ORG

APHA PRESS

AN IMPRINT OF AMERICAN PUBLIC HEALTH ASSOCIATION